By the same author:

Making The Transition To A Macrobiotic Diet

Our Food, Our Future

An Introduction To

MACROBIOTICS

A Beginner's Guide To The Natural Way Of Health

by
Carolyn
Heidenry

Aladdin Press
Boston

Published by Aladdin Press, 318 Harvard St., Suite 10, Brookline, MA 02146
ISBN: 0-916607-00-3
Library of Congress Catalog Card Number: 84-70161
Manufactured in the United States of America
Illustrations by Kathryn Lloyd
Cover design: Arts & Letters, Inc.
First edition: May 1984

DISTRIBUTOR:

Redwing Book Co.
44 Linden Street
Brookline MA 02146
617-738-4664

Acknowledgements

I would like to offer very special thanks to Paolo Antognetti for the many ways in which he helped to bring this book into being—from the moral support and encouragement he provided throughout its laborious revisions to the very capable editorial assistance he contributed. I am particularly grateful to him for the faith and confidence he has expressed in this book by becoming its publisher.

Table of Contents

Preface

Several purposes prompted the writing of this introduction to macrobiotics. Most important among them was the pressing need that exists for a brief and easily understood explanation of the macrobiotic diet. It is hoped that this book will assist in alleviating this need by helping to acquaint readers with the basic principle of yin and yang.

A glance at the contents will suffice to show that this brief introduction to what was once a traditional way of health in the Orient cannot, of course, be considered a comprehensive treatment of the myriad interrelationships between diet and health. In the following chapters I have only briefly touched upon the various ways in which foods can affect our health. Obviously, such an abbreviated presentation of this deep and centuries-old study carries with it great limitations. For reducing this comprehensive understanding of food to a few pages of practical information may, in some instances, subject it to misinterpretation or incorrect application. As the saying goes—"a little learning is a dangerous thing". However, it may, nonetheless, be justified by the acute need for a popularized introduction to this essential information, and from these first slender shoots of comprehension a deeper understanding may grow.

Perhaps the best service this book can render is to be a door for the reader—an entry point to further study about this traditional Oriental way of health. Other books will serve as the real teachers of this wisdom, written by those who understand it deeply and more fully. But even wisdom can be of little value when people cannot readily understand its substance or core. Therefore, this book was written with the hope that it would enable readers to understand the simple principle that is the essence of macrobiotics and to comprehend the great value it has for their lives.

In the West we have, unquestionably, learned much about ourselves and the world we live in. In science and technology we have reached heights once undreamed of. Yet somehow, in spite of these great advancements, a fundamental understanding of how foods affect the human organism has eluded us for centuries. The re-discovery of this knowledge in the East, its subsequent refinement, and its introduction to the West, now portend to initiate the most significant advance in our understanding of human nature yet seen in our entire history.

It will seem strange to some, no doubt, that this discovery is being heralded not by the usual sources from whom a major breakthrough might be expected—the scientists, doctors, researchers and leading experts of our day—but rather by a much younger and less prominent segment of our society. But as history shows, America is not a country that always opts for a conventional course of action. Consistent with this pattern, and unlikely as it may seem, it is the youth of America who are leading the burgeoning revolution in wholistic healthcare. We who are turning to the traditional healing arts of the East have recognized that while modern medicine is still searching for clues, traditional (Asian) medicine long ago found the answers. As a result of the beneficial changes tradi-

tional healthcare has made in our own lives, we are recommending it to others as a solution to the problems of widespread disease and social disorder now permeating our society. Sensing a way out of the maze of modern dilemmas confronting us, we dare to point the way towards a new and deeper understanding of health and a general regeneration of our culture.

It is important to state here that many of us, both young and old, who have had the good fortune to learn about the macrobiotic way of health owe what we know to a small group of individuals from Japan, where this forgotten wisdom was resurrected. Among them are the late George Ohsawa, his wife Lima Ohsawa, Michio and Aveline Kushi, Shizuko Yamamoto, Herman and Cornelia Aihara, Alcan and Hisako Yamaguchi, Hideo Ohmori, Clim Yoshimi, Toshi Kawaguchi, and Michiko Ogawa.

There is one member of this group, however, whose tireless efforts have clearly been exceptional in educating people around the world on the macrobiotic way of health. Through his books and seminars, guidance and counseling, discoveries and perceptions, many thousands of people have been relieved of their sufferings and given a second chance at a healthy and normal life. To him, Michio Kushi, this book is respectfully dedicated. With this dedication goes the hope that his contribution to America's health and future will one day be recognized and fully acknowledged with deepest gratitude. Considering both past and present attitudes towards Eastern medicine, it seems unlikely that this will occur within the foreseeable future. But in time—and how close or distant a time no one can surmise—it will surely be seen that through his life and work, more than that of any other, the renewal of health and peace we dream of, may come to be.

C. Heidenry

An Introduction to
MACROBIOTICS

Let thy food be thy medicine, and thy medicine be thy food.

HIPPOCRATES

Cause and Effect

It is widely known and generally accepted today that the American diet is becoming hazardous to our health, loaded down as it is with excessive amounts of cholesterol, saturated fats, refined sugar and chemical additives. Less agreement prevails, however, on what kind of diet provides the maximum benefits to our health. This may be due, in part, to the fact that we have not yet been successful in clearly identifying which dietary elements cause specific diseases[1] and which promote sound health. This basic connection—between dietary habits and their correlating effects (whether positive or negative)—has remained for centuries an unfathomed mystery.

Surprising as it may seem, in view of the massive search underway for cures to the diseases which plague us, the fundamental key to the colossal question of *which foods cause disease and which restore health* was discovered centuries ago in Asia. This key consists of a basic understanding of how the human body is affected, for better or worse, by various kinds of foods—*the raw material out of which it is continuously constructed.*

As this key or 'code' was more extensively deciphered, it was developed into a systematized body of knowledge and a better understanding of the role of food gradually evolved. Oriental doctors traditionally utilized this understanding of food to treat various kinds of health problems. However, in order to find a cure for a disorder, they first sought to find its cause—its source within an individual's diet. In other words they went directly to the heart of the matter to discover the reason why a problem developed. For sickness was not perceived as something which drops randomly out of the sky on hapless individuals, but rather as a condition which is produced by specific causes.

This traditional cause approach to healing is opposite to our modern cure approach, which aims primarily at the eradication or suppression of troublesome symptoms instead of seeking a deeper understanding of disease. Perhaps this is why more than a billion dollars worth of research annually fails to produce a cure for cancer. For no matter how much money is spent and no matter how much research is done, without an understanding of this cause-and-effect relationship, we can only engage in futile warfare against cancer and other diseases with an artillery of drugs, radiation and surgery. If we concern ourselves solely with the relief or removal of painful symptoms, whatever success we achieve will only be temporary. This is because, sooner or later, the original cause of a disorder, if not withdrawn, will once more begin to accumulate and eventually erupt. The cause approach is, therefore, the more sound approach, for once the source of a particular disorder is known, the cure[2] is automatically indicated—i.e. the elimination (or reduction) of the offending substances from the individual's diet.

For many centuries in parts of Asia, doctors gently yet effectively treated health problems by simply adjusting their patients' diets. This method of treatment not only relieves the symptoms of a disorder over a period of time, but also actually heals the organ or area of the body that is afflicted. This natural way of healing relies upon the body's remarkable capacity to repair itself when given the means to do so—that is, when given balanced, natural, whole foods.

The dietary system known as macrobiotics[3] is the embodiment and further refinement of this discovery which originated in China some thousands of years ago. Due to the successive efforts of several Japanese[4] in resurrecting and refining this knowledge, it is now being made available to the modern world. Macrobiotics, which is actually a very refined understanding of natural law, especially as it pertains to the human body, delineates the mechanism by which food influences our physical and mental state. As well, it defines the particular properties of various foods and whether they adversely or positively affect human health, both in general and with regard to specific diseases.

Macrobiotics is also a wholistic system of nutrition, which means that it takes into account the effect of food on our whole or entire organism—the physical, mental and emotional—for all are bound together. It includes both the interrelation and interaction between mind, body and food, a view of human nature unfamiliar to those of us who have considered the body and mind to be separate entities, little affected by what we eat.

Sensitive observation of the subtle changes that take place in the body's system subsequent to the consumption and absorption of various foods and liquids helped to create this refined dietary system. But in addition to the study of food and health, macrobiotics is actually a much broader body of knowledge—it is a comprehensive understanding of Nature itself in the largest sense of the word.[5] However, at its present stage of development, the study of macrobiotics is primarily focused on *the ways Nature generates change in the body through the means of food.*

Macrobiotics is necessarily a very practical system, based on the day-to-day art or practice of cooking healthy meals. Once the basic effects of foods were perceived and systematically organized, a healthful diet was developed from this advanced comprehension. In addition to a basic general diet, special recipes are utilized, when needed, to assist in relieving various types of disorders in the body. Through these means—simple natural, wholesome foods—pathological conditions can be gradually alleviated. This takes place through a slower, more natural process rather than via faster but more violent measures, such as surgery. This rare utilization of food is a sensitive art, light years away from our relatively primitive understanding of diet and its effect on health.

The word macrobiotics was chosen in an attempt to appropriately name this deep understanding of Nature. MACRO, meaning great, and BIOS, meaning life, join together to mean the great (view of) life. Macrobiotics has also been variously interpreted as the way of health and longevity, the great art of life and the ancient art of health. However, the word "macrobiotics" is simply the modern name for what originally was the study of how food and other natural influences affect us.[6] This unique understanding of health was the basis of Oriental medicine in various regions of the Far East, particularly in China and Japan, until the West appeared on the horizon with its tantalizing technology. As the East rushed to embrace the irresistible western 'magic,' the wisdom of generations was abandoned.[7] Traditional Oriental medicine faded and was forgotten in the overall race for technological parity, for they incorrectly assumed our medicine, which was rudimentary, to be on a par with our technology, which was advanced.

Now fortunately re-discovered, this traditional diet and way of health is being introduced to the modern world. It is based on a single simple principle, one which may be applied not only to the area of food and health, but to all other fields of study as well for it is a basic law of Nature. This book, however, does not address the many other possible applications of this principle, but rather concerns itself with its most timely and critical application—food and its influence on human health. Through relatively simple in theory, the diversified interplay of this principle in Nature can be a life time study. However, its core or essence is easy to perceive and understand, once it has been pointed out.

These are the eternal laws governing all phenomena . . . . visible and invisible . . . past and future.

MICHIO KUSHI

The Basic Principle

It was known from ancient times, then, in many parts of the world[8] that within the changing cycles and seasons of the earth an *order* existed—a particular pattern by which Nature, in all of her manifestations, moves. In observing this order, this grand design of Nature, we can perceive that *all energy in the universe moves in one of two basic, and opposite, directions.* This is why our world is composed of contrasting opposites . . . . . winter and summer, night and day, male and female. This pattern of contrasting opposites can be seen in every aspect of the universe, for all of Nature is influenced by these two fundamental energy patterns.

Generations of observation by ancient scholars confirmed the conclusion that without exception everything in the known universe is affected by this natural pattern or design of Nature, including human beings, plants, animals, minerals, and of course, the foods we eat. Both the vegetable kingdom (grains, fruits, vegetables, seeds and nuts) and the animal kingdom (mammals, fowl, and fish) are affected by these two primary energies which possess opposite and complementary qualities, as outlined below. The Chinese called them YIN and YANG (pronounced een and yähn). In order to write about them, it is necessary to borrow these two names for we have no words in our vocabulary as yet by which to call them.

Some foods were thought to be more affected by YANG influences, while other foods were considered to be more affected by YIN influences. YIN foods and YANG foods are opposite in their nature and in their fundamental qualities and, as a result, *in their effects on us when we eat them.* Both kinds of foods, however, are good for us and both are essential for life and growth.

The way in which different foods were categorized as either YIN or YANG was according to the qualities and characteristics each possesses. Every food has *both* YIN and YANG characteristics (for YIN and YANG always exist in combination with each other) but one influence or the other will always predominate. In other words, there is nothing which is neutral. If the majority of a food's characteristics are YANG, then that food is considered YANG, for that is the influence that predominates, and that is the *effect* that will predominate when we eat it. Generally, foods can be described by at least several of the following characteristics of one type or the other *(though not every characteristic will necessarily apply in every case.)*

YANG FOODS ARE:	YIN FOODS ARE:
More **small** or **compact** in size,	More **expanded** or **large** in size,
More **hard** or dense in texture,	More **soft** or less dense in texture,
More **dry** than moist,	More **moist** than dry,

More **thick** or heavy in weight,
More **salty** or **bitter** in taste,
More **round** in shape,
More **tight** in structure or composition,
Lower in potassium,
Thriving in **cooler weather** or climates.

More **thin** or light in weight,
More **sweet** or **sour** in taste,
More **long** in shape,
More **loose** in structure or composition,
Higher in potassium,
Thriving in **warmer weather** or climates.

AMONG ANIMALS, MORE YANG ANIMALS ARE:
More **active,**
More **aggressive,** or
Faster-moving.

AMONG ANIMALS, MORE YIN ANIMALS ARE:
More **inactive,**
More **passive,** or
Slower-moving.

An example of how these different qualities are present in our foods may be seen in the following comparison.

Watermelon is a more YIN food. It is *large* and *expanded* in size, *soft* in texture and full of *moisture*. It is also a food which is *high in potassium* and one which *grows in warmer weather*. Buckwheat is a very different type of food, i.e., it is a more YANG food. Buckwheat is *small* and *compact* in size, relatively *hard* and *dense* in texture, and more *dry* than moist. It is also *low in potassium* and *grows well in colder weather*.

Therefore, we can see that watermelon has many YIN characteristics while buckwheat possesses many YANG characteristics. Were we to eat watermelon everyday for an extended period of time we would eventually begin to experience some YIN symptoms. We might develop a runny nose or frequent urination (two of the body's ways of eliminating excess *water*) or we might develop a red color on our cheeks from *expanding* blood capillaries. The reverse would be true if we were to eat buckwheat everyday for an extended period of time. We would eventually begin to develop some YANG symptoms. This might appear as a tightness or inability to relax, a sustained feeling of tension or some other indication of the too *contracted* condition we were developing.

In either case the degree and frequency of the effects that appeared would be, in part, affected by what other kinds of foods we were eating and the quantity of watermelon or buckwheat we consumed. Both of these foods are wholesome, of course, when eaten as part of a rounded diet. Since they have relatively moderate qualities *their effects are also relatively moderate,* even when taken in excess.[9]

For there are some foods which are moderately YIN or YANG and other foods which are extremely YIN or YANG. This is determined by various factors, but primarily by a food's original properties, and secondarily by the way it is cooked or processed, as will be explained. These more extreme foods possess extreme qualities which make them unsuitable to eat, for this cause-and-effect process, as just shown with the example of watermelon and buckwheat, becomes magnified many times over. In other words, *the more extreme the food, the more extreme the effect.*

We may not be aware of it, but we automatically try to keep a general balance in our diet between these YIN and YANG types of foods. This helps us maintain an equilibrium in our bodies that keeps us healthy. If we eat only YIN foods we instinctively begin to crave YANG foods, and vice versa, for this is Nature's way of maintaining a balance. When we eat a steak dinner, for example, (meat is an extreme YANG food) we usually also have a sweet dessert or a soft drink or an alcoholic beverage—which are extreme YIN foods. At the very least we have vegetables, fruit or salad (which are more moderately YIN foods). If we took only the steak—without sweets or alcohol or at least vegetables or fruits—we would begin to feel uncomfortable and unsatisfied, as if something were missing. In a little while we would want to have a soda, or perhaps an ice cream, or some other YIN type of food. Similarly, in the morning we eat an extreme YANG food—eggs—together with an extreme YIN food—orange juice. At lunch we choose a hamburger—extreme YANG—and a soft drink—extreme YIN. In the evening, when watching television, we sip a beer or soda—YIN—while snacking on something salty and dry—YANG—such as popcorn or pretzels. Our bodies constantly demand this balance, and thus we automatically combine these two opposite types of foods in our diet everyday, whether we are conscious of it or not.

There are many examples in the cuisine of every country which show this tendency to maintain a balance of YIN and YANG by combining two opposite types of foods. Some cuisines accomplish this more successfully than others, but no society (or individual) eats only YANG foods or only YIN foods—that is, not without ill effects. If we attempt to do so for any length of time a strong desire for an opposite kind of food will arise. Should we persist in eating only one type of food—YIN or YANG—or if we are forced by an unusual situation to persist, the result, sooner or later, is sickness. Depending on the foods involved and the length of time they are consumed, eventually death can occur.[10]

In most people, the instinct for balance quickly surfaces, usually without their realizing it, when they have eaten too much of any one type of food. Our internal systems may, in fact, be likened to a see-saw that can easily go too far up (too YIN) or too far down (too YANG), depending on whether we eat too many of these YIN foods or too many of these YANG foods. The more we know about YIN and YANG, the easier it becomes to balance this see-saw, for this enables us to more safely control this process instead of blindly allowing it to control us. It is much more difficult to maintain an appropriate balance of YIN and YANG when we consume more extreme foods, for then this see-saw begins to swing out of control. When we choose foods which are more moderate it becomes easier to maintain a relatively balanced condition in our bodies. Understanding this interaction of YIN and YANG may seem difficult at first, but like a new game, once the 'rules' are learned and a little practice acquired, one can eventually become adept at using this valuable tool to restore and maintain health and well-being.

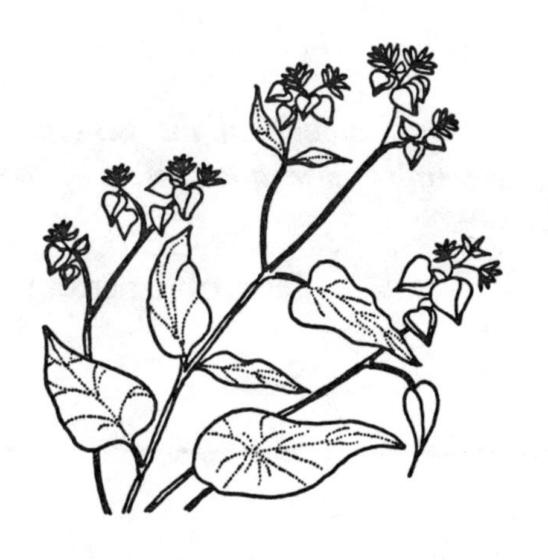

Buckwheat

If we only knew enough, all diseases could be prevented and cured through proper nutrition.

TOM SPIES
Dean of American Nutritionists

Disease As Imbalance

We see, therefore, how problems can arise when we consume extreme foods for these foods are so yin or so yang that they are beyond what most people can safely tolerate. Extreme foods are not as smoothly handled by the body and various kinds of disorders eventually result from their effects or their accumulation. When these foods are consumed in large quantities, or on a very frequent basis, the incidence of physical and mental disorders in a society begins to increase markedly. When they constitute the major part of our diet, as they unfortunately do today, degenerative disease becomes widespread, as our recent health statistics show.

This is because when we consume either very yin or very yang foods over a period of time, we ourselves tend to become very yin or very yang as well; which means that in subtle and curious ways the eater begins to resemble that which is eaten. As stated in the well-known remark—"you are what you eat," this happens because *we tend to absorb the characteristics possessed by the foods we consume*. So when we frequently eat extreme foods, we gradually begin to acquire an extreme condition, an unbalanced condition, and this state we call sickness or disease.

This cause-and-effect process is one of the main branches of macrobiotic study. Accordingly, various diseases have been classified as the result of either an excess of yin foods or an excess of yang foods. By determining which particular foods produce a disorder and then by eliminating those foods from one's diet (or in some cases by only reducing the amount taken), specific diseases can be prevented and often alleviated. When a disease or disorder is caused by an excess of yang foods, obviously it is necessary to decrease one's intake of yang foods, while somewhat increasing the intake of moderately yin foods which help restore a state of balance to the body. In addition, a standard macrobiotic diet should be consumed in order to provide the kind of continuous balanced nourishment the body can use to slowly reconstruct itself.[11] In the case of a sickness produced by extreme yin foods it is necessary to reverse this procedure and lessen one's intake of yin foods, supplanting them with moderately yang foods. Once again it is necessary to consume a basic macrobiotic diet, which aids in neutralizing the disorder and generally contributes to the maintainance of health. In this way balance is gradually restored to the body, as it absorbs these more moderate, less extreme foods.

Two other important factors necessary to the alleviation of a disorder are the correct preparation of meals, which should not be carelessly selected or cooked, but prepared according to correct procedures; and secondly, the adoption of a healthful lifestyle, which primarily consists of adequate physical exercise and thorough chewing of one's food.

So from the macrobiotic perspective health is understood as a state where a harmonious balance between yin and yang is maintained. Optimum health, therefore, is achieved by eating a balanced diet, one which is neither extremely yin nor extremely yang, but composed of more moderate type foods. Though this is an oversimplification for the sake of clarity, this was the basic principle involved in the formation of the macrobiotic diet.

Since most disorders arise from a state of imbalance *created by what we put into our bodies,* (whether it be in the form of food, beverages, drugs, or even through breathing toxic fumes, etc.) we can protect ourselves by selecting foods and beverages which are more beneficial to our health and by avoiding foods and beverages which tend to produce illness. Our present dietary trend is to eat any kind of food we please year after year after year. When trouble eventually develops at some point, we haul our body to the doctor, the way we take our car to the mechanic, expecting it to be repaired in a similar fashion. Doctors do their best, even installing 'new parts' recently, through heart and liver transplants. But by placing what really amounts to the entire responsibility for our health on our doctor's shoulders, we create a dangerous situation; for doctors cannot undo with a few operations or drugs damage we have allowed to build up for years. Now, by acquiring a knowledge of *how to eat,* we will be able to take better preventive measures in caring for our health than has previously been possible. By understanding that foods transfer their innate properties to the eater, we can learn to detect the patterns of how physical and mental disorders are created.

Disorders can manifest in many different ways even within persons of the same family, for no two individuals behave in exactly the same manner. No two people consume exactly the same quantity or exactly the same type of foods; nor do they exercise the same amount (i.e. discharge the food eaten in the same way) and no two are born with identical constitutions—a factor that determines one's inherent strengths and weaknesses. Accordingly, depending on these varying factors—constitution, exercise, quantity and type of foods eaten—as well as other factors such as age and sex, an individual may be predisposed to one type of health problem, yet remain free of another. Understanding the effects of extreme yin and extreme yang foods, and the influence of these secondary factors, sheds light at last on how the human body operates and makes visible the reasons why various disorders afflict some people while not others.

Similarly, mental and emotional problems are also often the result of an incorrect diet. As the ancient Romans said 'mens sana in corpore sana"—a sound mind in a sound body. They understood the link between the two and knew that the body and mind are not separate entities, as we moderns have presumed. In macrobiotic principles, this idea is expressed as "physiology precedes and determines psychology".[12] As we know, the body develops *before* the mind. Cells become egg and sperm, which then become an embryo, which eventually forms into a fetus, which is born as an infant. In time, the infant grows into a child who gradually develops into an adolescent and then a full-grown adult. From the time the body is fully formed at birth, consciousness slowly awakens over the years; the mind begins to expand and develop as the body slows down and completes its growth.

This mind is dependent on the body for its formation and growth,[13] so much a part, so intertwined is it with the body. What we feed the body, therefore, is as important for the mind as it is for the growing body, as we know from studies done on hyperkinetic children. These studies show that abnormal personalities and behavior can be returned to normal when the food consumed by these children is untainted with various chemicals and additives.[14] This indicates that the condition of the mind is dependent upon the condition of the body. Mental problems cannot only be seen as simply "psychological" problems to be dealt with separately from the body, as if they were somehow isolated from the rest of an individual's being and substance.

According to the macrobiotic perspective, many mental abnormalities are logical and predictable psychological consequences of unbalanced *physical* conditions. The great importance of this fact is the realization that relief from this type of suffering may be obtained, in time, through appropriate dietary alteration. By correctly adjusting the food being consumed and absorbed by mentally ill individuals, the vast majority of mental problems can be alleviated in the same way as physical disorders.

We know that every disease, mental or physical, has a particular set of symptoms by which it is recognized. This is because every disease is the result of a particular cause, or set of causes, which always produce similar specific effects. There are types of cancer, for instance, which are produced by the overconsumption of extreme yang foods—such as meat and eggs, and there are types of cancer which are produced by the overconsumption of extreme yin foods—such as ice cream and sugar. The same holds true for heart disease and other kinds of major and minor illnesses, from diabetes and muscular dystrophy to acne and headaches.

The best and most thorough treatment of this subject (disorders—their cause and alleviation) may be found in the works of Michio Kushi[15], including numerous case histories of people who have cleansed themselves of various diseases through eating a macrobiotic diet. However the following is a partial list of various disorders caused by excessive consumption of extreme foods over a long period of time.

EXCESS YIN FOODS	*EXCESS YANG FOODS*	*EXCESS YIN and YANG FOODS*
Leukemia	Jaundice	Arteriosclerosis
Meningitis	Gout	Hepatitis
Colitis	Duodenal Ulcers	Uremia
Epilepsy	Liver Cancer	Gallstones
Emphysema	Tongue Cancer	Breast Cancer
Diabetes	Lung Cancer	Kidney Cancer
Asthma	Pancreatic Cancer	Uterine Cancer
Skin Cancer	Colon Cancer	Bladder Cancer
Hypersensitivity	Muscular Dystrophy	Schizophrenia
Nervousness	Anger	
	Paranoia	

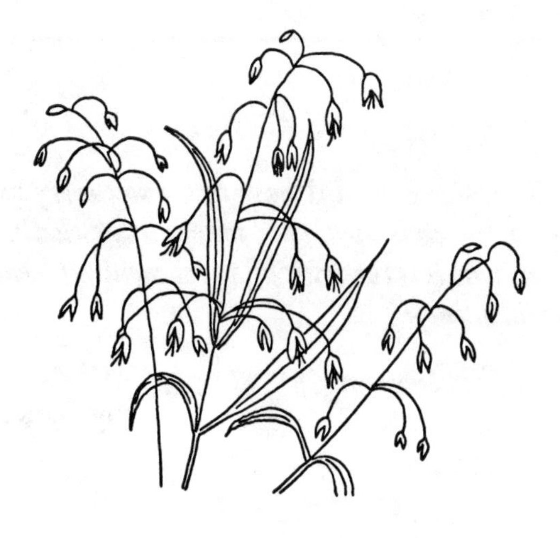

Oats

And God said, Behold, I have given you every herb bearing seed, which is upon the face of all the earth, and every tree in which is the fruit of a tree yielding seed: to you it shall be for meat.

GENESIS 1:29
King James Bible

The Macrobiotic Diet

Which foods are of a moderate type and which are of an extreme type? Which produce more detrimental effects and which produce more beneficial effects? The chart on page 34 & 35 shows the classification of foods according to yin and yang. On the left and right sides of the chart are those foods which are the more extreme types (and which consequently produce extreme effects in our systems), while towards the center of the chart are those foods which are more moderate types, neither excessively yin or yang in their original properties.[16]

The macrobiotic diet has been designed around the central range of foods on the chart. These more balanced foods consist basically of wholegrains, fresh vegetables, fish (which can be optional), beans and legumes, seeds, nuts, fruits and soy products. These are the foods which may be safely consumed on a daily basis.[17] They also provide all the nutrients required to maintain good health—proteins, carbodydrates, minerals and vitamins.[18]

Within the macrobiotic diet there are moderately yin

foods and moderately yang foods, but not the extremely yin or extremely yang foods at the far sides of the chart. Many traditional cultures throughout the world instinctively followed this general dietary pattern, avoiding extreme types of foods. They minimized the use of meat, alcohol and sweets, and emphasized the use of grains and vegetables. Until recent times there has been a natural pattern of *grain* as the principal food in most parts of the world, except in very cold regions where fish or meat is required to withstand the harsh weather (for extreme climates require more extreme foods).

More than any other food, grain has traditionally been the central dietary element on which mankind has depended. In many Oriental countries it was rice that was traditionally the center of every meal—brown rice until modern food processing techniques were invented that removed its precious nutrients. The Japanese even went so far as to feel that a meal without rice was not really a meal. In the Middle East there was extensive use of both wheat and rice and their many derivatives such as couscous and bulghur. In Europe and Russia, wheat, barley, oats, rye and buckwheat played major roles in the development and sustenance of these civilizations (though less so in recent times), while in the Americas, corn or maize was the most widely used grain. Most traditional cultures have centered their diets around these foods keeping a general ratio of grain as the principal food, with vegetables, beans, fish and meat as secondary dishes.[19]

America, however, has drastically lowered its consumption of grains over the years. What grain *is* consumed now, is often taken in such highly processed forms as white bread, cold cereals, corn syrup and so forth; these extremely refined foods do not furnish the strong sustaining nourishment that is provided by wholegrains. Since we no longer consume the most important element of sound nutrition—wholegrain—chaotic food habits and behavior predictably result. This is because by eating contrary to dietary order we gradually become "out of order" ourselves, incorrectly functioning in various ways. Therefore to restore health and order to our society, it is necessary to restore wholegrain to its central role in our diet.

This is why a macrobiotic meal is always centered around a wholegrain food as the base on which to build the rest of the meal. This grain dish is usually accompanied by a hot nourishing soup, a protein food such as fish, tofu or beans, and several kinds of freshly cooked vegetables. Roasted seeds or nuts and sea greens help complement the meal. In addition, fresh fruit or a naturally-sweetened dessert may also be included if desired. These are the standard components of macrobiotic meals which may be prepared in an international variety of ways using styles of cooking as different as American, French, Chinese, Japanese, Mexican, Italian, and Indian (etc.), according to individual preference. These simple staples—grains, vegetables, beans, seeds and fruits have sustained many great nations throughout history, and can be fashioned into an extensive and pleasing array of menus. So neither variety nor flavor need be sacrificed in adopting a macrobiotic diet.

Recommended Foods

The following food groups explain in more detail the kinds of foods most often used in macrobiotic cuisine.

SOUPS

Many delicious soups can be made that greatly contribute to the satisfaction of a healthy diet. These range all the way from hearty bean soups to light delicate broths, and include vegetable soups, barley soups, noodle soups, fish chowders, vegetable purees, minestrone, and rich stews.

WHOLEGRAINS

This basic food of man has been cooked in as many ways as there are countries in the world. To name only a few there is Chinese-style fried rice, Spanish-style shellfish and rice—*paella,* Middle Eastern *wheat pilaf* and *pita* bread, and Mexican *tortillas* and *tamales.* In addition there are various kinds of Italian corn and rice dishes such as *polenta* and *risotto,* and many kinds of wholegrain *pasta.* From India come the famous *puri* and *chapati* breads, and from Russia, the renowned black breads and *kasha* dishes. Other well-known grain dishes include Moroccan *couscous,* delicate French buckwheat *crepes,* Greek rice and grapeleaf rolls—*dolmados*—and the many rice and noodle dishes of Japan—*nori-maki, sushi, mochi, soba* and *udon.* And last but not least, there are South American corn dishes such as *arepas,* and the "all-American" foods that can be prepared with wholegrain flour—wheat, corn and rye breads, waffles and pancakes, biscuits, and muffins.

VEGETABLES

Vegetables of all kinds, including dark, nutritious leafy greens and hardy roots, are also adaptable to many different styles of preparation. They can be braised or sauted, stir-fried or steamed, baked or boiled, deep-fried, pickled, marinated or eaten raw. Unfortunately, vegetables do not always receive the proper attention or careful treatment that they deserve. In American cuisine they are often overcooked or canned or frozen. Most Oriental cooks and many European cooks treat their vegetables with more care, with the result that they have fresher, tastier and more appealing vegetable dishes.

SOYFOODS, BEANS AND VEGETABLE PROTEINS

There are many tasty varieties of beans and legumes that add variety and hearty nutrition to grain dishes and vegetable or soup recipes. In addition, there are many new soyfoods which are now making inroads into American cuisine. These include tofu (soy cheese), miso (soup-flavoring) and tempeh (soy meat). Another popular food is a product known as 'wheatmeat' which is a wheat gluten protein. Many of these foods are easily fashioned into soy 'burgers', pot pies, 'steaks' and 'cutlets'. They can be stewed, grilled or roasted just like meat. There is even tofu 'cheesecake', tofu 'quiche', soy 'sausage' and various kinds of dips and sandwich spreads. These traditional natural foods—tofu, wheatmeat, and tempeh are the versatile new wonder foods just arriving on the American scene and destined to make it big as the natural eater's protein.

SEAGREENS

These vegetables, also called seaweed or sometimes sea vegetables, grow in the ocean and vary in flavor and appearance just as vegetables grown on the land do. They look and taste as different as cauliflower, carrots, corn and broccoli. Some are strong in taste and some are mild, while others have a spicy flavor. They can be ground into a dry powder and sprinkled on foods like salt and pepper or they may be eaten as a vegetable dish like carrots or peas. Frequently they are cooked and then served chilled with a dressing as part of a mixed salad.

SEAFOOD AND FISH

A good quality animal protein, fish and seafood are plentiful in many varieties and may be prepared as either a succulent grill or poached in a delicate sauce. They can also be pan-fried or deep-fried, broiled or barbequed, marinated or baked, and even eaten raw, Japanese-style, in a delicate and beautifully arranged dish known as sashimi.

SEEDS AND NUTS

Nutritious, protein-packed seeds and nuts (lightly roasted) enhance meals with their excellent flavor and also serve as wholesome between-meal snacks.

FRUITS

Fresh or dried, fruits lend their charms to an abundance of naturally-sweet desserts from whips, gelatins and puddings to pies, cakes, cookies and jams.

NATURAL SWEETENERS

Other wholesome natural sweeteners include 'made-from-grain' sweeteners such as barley-malt or rice-syrup, in addition to maple syrup and fruit concentrates which are available at most good natural food stores.

SEASONINGS

Oil—Animal fats such as lard and butter are not used in macrobiotic cooking due to their animal source. Instead, good quality, unrefined oils are recommended such as sesame oil, sunflower oil and safflower oil, as well as corn oil and soybean oil. Expeller-pressed oils from a reputable natural food company are preferred over those extracted by chemical solvents.

Salt—Free of the additives that are now used in processing table salt—which is a highly concentrated form of sodium—white, unrefined sea salt is preferred, because it is obtained by natural methods from sea water and retains important trace minerals.[20]

Spices—Instead of strong spices, which are yin due to their stimulant qualities, only mild seasonings and flavorings are used in macrobiotic cooking, except very occasionally. These include parsley, scallion, ginger, tamari soy sauce, miso soup-flavoring, rice vinegar, and sesame salt among many others.

BEVERAGES

Mild teas and grain coffees (coffee-like beverages made from roasted, powdered grains) are recommended over strong teas and coffee which are very yin. Fruit juices are substituted for soft drinks which are avoided altogether. Alcoholic beverages are not recommended, but if desired, very moderate amounts of a good quality, non-chemicalized beer or rice wine are preferable.

Variety and Flexibility

With such abundance and variety, no lack of flavor or satisfaction need occur when eating a macrobiotic diet. Those who eat natural foods, which means whole and unprocessed, the way Nature made them, reap the best of both worlds; they enjoy a wide spectrum of the earth's harvest without sacrificing their health, the unfortunate result of so many other diets. Natural foods combine deliciously in the hands of a good cook and the only limitations in flavor or appeal that result are those which arise from the limited skills of the cook. This is one reason why it is important to study the art of macrobiotic cooking very well.

But selecting one's food from this moderate range of foods *in itself* does not automatically guarantee perfect health. Because even wholesome foods can be unhealthful when eaten to excess or out of proportion with each other. So it is important to remember that these foods are beneficial only when eaten in sufficient variety and when properly cooked.

Another factor to take into account in selecting one's diet is the amount of activity or work one engages in. This is important because those who are involved in manual labor or sports activities naturally require a larger quantity of food and liquid and some animal protein of good quality such as fish. Those who have less physically-active occupations obviously require lesser quantities of food and liquid and less animal protein.

Age is also a factor worthy of consideration. Children, for example, being small and active (i.e. yang) need *very little salt,* for salt is also yang. When given too much salt children can become overly yang quite easily. They require good quality yin foods to grow (yin is expansive in direction and therefore assists in growth) such as a little more liquid, more vegetable proteins, and good quality sweets, in addition to regular (low-salt) macrobiotic meals. Infants should be given no salt at all for they are very small and yang, and salt can be dangerous for them. Their natural food at this very yang stage of their life is sweet mother's milk (yin) for Nature is always making balance.[21]

Since family members often have individual differences a good cook will provide a sufficient range of foods to allow everyone to meet their various requirements.

Ideally this should be a natural instinctive way of satisfying everyone's needs, not a complicated mental process. Of course, the success of this process is almost entirely dependent on the daily provision of good, hearty wholesome meals of sufficient variety. This really means, then, that the health of a family is largely in the hands of the cook.

Therefore, it can be seen that a macrobiotic diet is not a fixed regimen of set menus, which could not possibly be appropriate for every type of person in the world or for every type of climate that exists. Instead, the macrobiotic diet is centered around a basic dietary pattern (considered most beneficial for the human body) that can be flexibly adapted to our changing activities and individual differences.

As other factors change in our lives, our age, our activity, or the seasons, etc., we can, through well-balanced meals, adjust our food in response to these changing factors and remain healthy. With slight alterations from one to another, we can consciously create the meals that are most appropriate for our changing needs, while still remaining in accord with basic guidelines that safeguard our health. This permits us to maximize the positive influence of wholesome foods and minimize the negative influence of unwholesome foods, using the *flexible* but *always centered,* macrobiotic diet.[22]

YIN-YANG FOOD

EXTREME YANG FOODS

MODERATE

VARIOUS CHEMICALS & DRUGS	EGGS	MEAT	POULTRY[1]	FISH & SEAFOOD[2]	FISH & SEAFOOD	WHOLEGRAINS[3]		SEEDS & NUTS	BEANS & VEGETABLE PROTEINS
For example:	*From poultry, or from fish, such as:*	Beef	Chicken	Bluefish	Carp	Barley	Bread	Almonds	Aduki Beans
Insulin	Caviar	Lamb	Duck	Salmon	Clams	Brown Rice	Corn Meal	Filberts	Black Beans
Thyroxin	Hen's eggs	Mutton	Goose	Swordfish	Cod	Buckwheat	Couscous	Peanuts	Chickpeas
		Pork	Pheasant	Tuna	Flounder	Corn	Cracked Wheat	Pecans	Kidney Beans
		Rabbit	Turkey		Haddock	Millet	Noodles	Poppy Seeds	Lentils
		Veal			Halibut	Oats	Oatmeal	Pumpkin Seeds	Lima Beans
		Wild game			Herring	Rye	Pasta	Squash Seeds	Navy Beans
					Oysters	Wheat	Sweet Rice	Sunflower Seeds	Pinto Beans
					Red Snapper			Walnuts	Soybeans
					Scallops				Split Peas
					Shrimp				Tempeh "Soymeat"
					Smelt				Tofu "Soycheese"
					Sole				Wheatmeat
					Trout				

The above chart is not meant to be an exhaustive list of all foods consumed (or avoided) on the macrobiotic diet, but just large enough to show the general range of food classification from yin to yang. In addition, precise classification cannot be indicated since the quality of foods may be changed during the cooking process.

Note: In the macrobiotic diet, all foods recommended as beneficial mean beneficial when consumed as one element of a varied and rounded diet. Any food which is consumed exclusively, without other essential nutrients, can become unhealthful.

LASSIFICATION

OODS

EXTREME YIN FOODS

SEA REENS	VEGETABLES[4]		FRUITS	SWEETENERS	TROPICAL FRUITS & NUTS	DAIRY FOODS	SWEETENERS[7]	STIMULANTS	VARIOUS CHEMICALS & DRUGS
ar Agar	*Roots/Stem*	*Greens*	*Fresh & Dried*	Barley Malt	Bananas	Butter[5]	Corn Syrup	Alcohol	*For example:*
ame	Burdock	Broccoli	Apples	Fruit Juice	Brazil Nuts	Cheese[6]	Chocolate	Spices	Aspirin
lse	Carrots	Brussel Sprouts	Apricots	Maple Syrup	Cashews	Cream	Honey		Cortizone
iki	Cauliflower	Cabbage	Blueberries	Rice Syrup	Coconut	Ice Cream	Molasses		LSD
sh Moss	Daikon Radish	Carrot Tops	Cantelope		Figs	Mayonnaise	Saccharine		Marijuana
mbu	Onions	Celery	Cherries		Grapefruit	Milk	Sugar		
kabu	Parsnips	Chinese Cabbage	Chestnuts		Hazelnuts	Yogurt			
ri	Pumpkin	Chives	Grapes		Kiwi Fruit				
kame	Radishes	Collard Greens	Peaches		Mangoes				
	Rutebaga	Cucumbers	Pears		Oranges				
	Stringbeans	Daikon Tops	Plums		Papayas				
	Summer Squash (Crookneck, Pattipan, etc.)	Endive	Raisins		Pistachios				
	Turnip	Kale	Raspberries						
	Winter Squash (Acorn, Buttercup, Butternut, Hokkaido, Hubbard, etc.)	Leeks	Strawberries						
		Lettuce	Watermelon						
		Mustard Greens							
		Parsley							
		Peas							
		Scallions							
		Swiss Chard							
		Turnip Greens							
		Watercress							

1 Or other wild or domesticated fowl.

2 And all other red-fleshed or blue-skinned fish.

3 Products derived from *refined* grains, such as white bread or white rice, are *not* recommended.

4 Potatoes, tomatoes, eggplant and several other vegetables are not recommended because of their extreme yin characteristics, i.e., tropical origin, potassium content, etc.

5 Also margarine.

6 Several salty, well-aged cheeses, which are very yang rather than yin, such as brie, roquefort, etc. should also be avoided.

7 And all products containing any of these sweeteners — such as soft drinks, candy, pastries, etc.

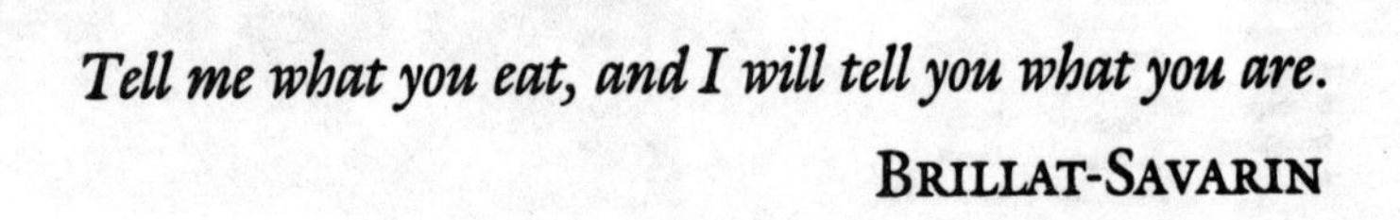

Tell me what you eat, and I will tell you what you are.

BRILLAT-SAVARIN

Nature's Designs

The macrobiotic diet is also in accord with various designs provided by Nature that indicate what our food should be. These designs, such as our teeth and digestive tract, as well as the seasonally-changing vegetation, all form a series of guideposts that show us what direction our diet should take.

Our Teeth

Every animal holds in its mouth a natural indication of the types of foods inherently suited to its species. Predatory animals, for instance, have sharp pointed teeth suitable for catching, holding and killing prey and tearing meat from bones. The role these animals play in keeping a balance in nature (i.e. certain groups of other animals from over-populating) makes meat their natural and proper food, and they are thus equipped with the kind of tools (teeth, claws, highly developed sense of smell, capacity for speed, etc.) necessary to obtain it, which human beings do not possess.

Grazing animals, on the other hand, have the molars and cutting teeth suitable for tearing grasses and plants from the ground and grinding them sufficiently for the digestive process to take place. In carnivorous animals meat is digested by enzymes in the stomach and need not be chewed. Plant foods, however, must be thoroughly masticated and mixed with the enzymes secreted in the mouth in order to be digested. The teeth of human beings consist primarily of molars and premolars and secondarily of incisors, whose purposes are to grind, chew and cut. This indicates that our main food should be from plant sources (such as grains, beans, vegetables, seeds, nuts, and so forth) which require grinding and chewing. We possess only four canine teeth, out of a total of thirty-two, which shows that meat or animal protein should be only a very small portion of our diet—not our main food.

Our Digestive Track

Similarly, the digestive track of predatory animals is suitable for the consumption of meat. Carnivores have a short digestive track to rapidly expell the toxic substances that result from the digestion of meat. Herbivores, on the other hand, have long digestive tracks *as do human beings,* which are suited to the slower assimilation process required for plant foods. It would obviously be unnatural and unhealthy for a carnivorous animal to try to obtain its sustenance from grass and foliage, and it would be just as abnormal for an herbivorous animal to try to eat flesh. Each has its place in Nature's plan and each has the appropriate digestive track and specialized tools in its mouth to act appropriately within the natural order into which all creatures are born.

As human beings, we are the most developed of all species, and so we can eat and survive on almost any type of food. In other words, we have the maximum ability to adapt to any circumstances or environment. However, some of the extreme foods we *can* eat to survive may sustain life, but at a price—the price being various detrimental effects to our health. But judging from our teeth and our long digestive track, it is clear that the majority of our food should be from the plant kingdom, while a small portion of our food may be from animal sources without disturbing our systems. Yet, born with these natural indicators, we ignore these important signs and eat as though we possess the teeth, claws and digestive track of carnivores.

The Climate We Live In

Another natural indicator of how we should eat may be seen in our environment. By observing what nature produces in any given climate and what thrives there, we can see the general types of foods which are appropriate for that region. The more extreme examples of the arctic and the tropics demonstrate this point very clearly. The foliage that grows in each of these two regions is very different, each kind responding to a specialized climate. In the extreme North, where the temperature is very cold (that is—very yin) the vegetation becomes stunted, contracted, tough and low to the ground (yang) in order to survive. Near the equator where it is very hot (that is—very yang) the vegetation grows tall, lush and expanded with wide leaves, large fruits and delicate flowers (yin). By developing qualities that are *opposite* to its environment vegetation 'balances' the climate and is thus able to survive; for in Nature, yin and yang are always balanced. So plants extensively adapt themselves in their attempt to thrive in specialized circumstances. This specialization occurs in many more subtle ways all over the world in response to varying climatic conditions, from the mountains to the plains to the sea. For each climate requires different qualities from plants and animals in order for them to survive. For example, the delicate, soft petals of jungle flowers could not withstand the harsh extremities of the North; and the polar bear would be most uncomfortable with his thick coat in the tropics.

When vegetation in hot, yang climates adapts by becoming very large and yin, and when vegetation in cold, yin climates adapts by becoming very small and yang, an important balance is being sought and achieved by Nature, one which should not go unheeded by us. Herbivorous animals in each area feed on the natural vegetation existing in their locale and thrive accordingly because *the qualities the plants have developed to thrive in that particular climate are transferred to the eater;* and in this way the animal is also able to comfortably thrive in the same climate as well. The animals of India and Africa consume the type of vegetation growing there and thrive comfortably under high temperatures. In the frozen arctic, the caribou and groundmice consume the sparse and contracted leaves, grasses, plants and seeds in their environment and also thrive because of their specialized diet. In each case, the animals adapt successfully to their environment by assimilating the local vegetation, a slow and gradual process which evolution has wondrously refined.

Only human beings confuse this natural order. By importing foods North and South, by consuming foods which grow to harmonize with a *different* climate we create further confusion and imbalance in our body chemistry. Our expertise and ability to roam the world and transport anything we find back to our original habitat, as well as our capacity to grow foods by using artificial methods, has brought us the wherewithal to turn Nature's balancing mechanism topsy-turvy, and undermine our health in the process.

The monkeys and giraffes of Africa do not import salty cheeses and canned meats to consume in their equatorial climate, nor do arctic rabbits order shipments of pineapples and bananas to nibble in their wintry hovels. Were any of them capable of such a feat they would soon become sick and die, unless well-equipped with central heating, air conditioning, medications and other artificial life supports. Rather, each eats within the range of foods nature has provided in its environment, and by doing so, maintains the right balance between its external environment and its internal system. This natural order protects them and keeps them healthy; it permits them to withstand the rigors of cold and heat just as the vegetation they eat is capable of doing. The principle underlying this perspective is that *environment creates its opposite, while food creates its similarity.*[23] So, though plants grow in ways opposite to their environment to balance the climate and thus survive, *when eaten* they produce effects similar to their own nature. Melons, cucumbers and lettuce (all yin) when eaten, produce cooling, yin effects similar to their own nature. Root vegetables, such as turnips, carrots and onions (more yang) produce more activating, warming, yang effects.

Therefore, to establish our own balance with Nature, it is important that we primarily eat foods which are grown in the environment in which we live. This means that the majority of the vegetables, grains, fruits, nuts, etc. which we eat should be grown preferably in our own region, or at least in the same general latitude or climate as the one in which we live. A person living in a temperate climate, therefore, should eat foods grown within a temperate region, rather than those imported from tropical climates.

The Changing Seasons

Seasonally there is a similar correlation. It used to be that summer fruits such as peaches, strawberries, and melons were eaten only when they ripened in the course of their natural cycle, during the warmer months of the year. With their cooling sweet juice and pulp they helped to balance the warmer seasons. Hardier fruits that stored well without decomposing (more yang) such as winter pears, apples and chestnuts, or fruits that could be dried—i.e. further yangized through contraction and elimination of water—were eaten over the colder months of the year. (Today we eat highly perishable fruits imported from tropical climates even in freezing weather.) When we do not tamper with Nature's cycles by artificial growing methods or by importing foods from vastly different climates, Nature provides the correct vegetables and fruits to harmonize with the changing seasons.[24] Grains, beans and seeds are staple foods for the whole year, indicated by their ability to store year-round without decomposing.

In very cold (yin) weather, or in cold regions of the world, food which best balances the environment should be consumed, i.e. food which is a little more yang. This means not only the local foods to be found there but also food which is well-cooked (fire is a yang factor) rather than food which is lightly cooked, or meals which include more fish or seafood, and dried fruits rather than fresh. In hot, yang weather or regions, the heat can be balanced with more yin foods, more uncooked foods, such as salad or raw fruit, as well as lighter styles of cooking, and less salt.

Eating a natural diet encompasses more than just eating natural foods, if we want to maintain good health. Good health demands that we acquire a basic understanding of the ways of Nature, her seasons and cycles, her "reasons" and designs. Understanding the natural order of the world makes it possible now for us to select the foods best suited to our environment. By using common sense and the natural signs offered by our teeth and digestive system, the climate we live in and the changing seasons, we can keep our health and remain in harmony with Nature.

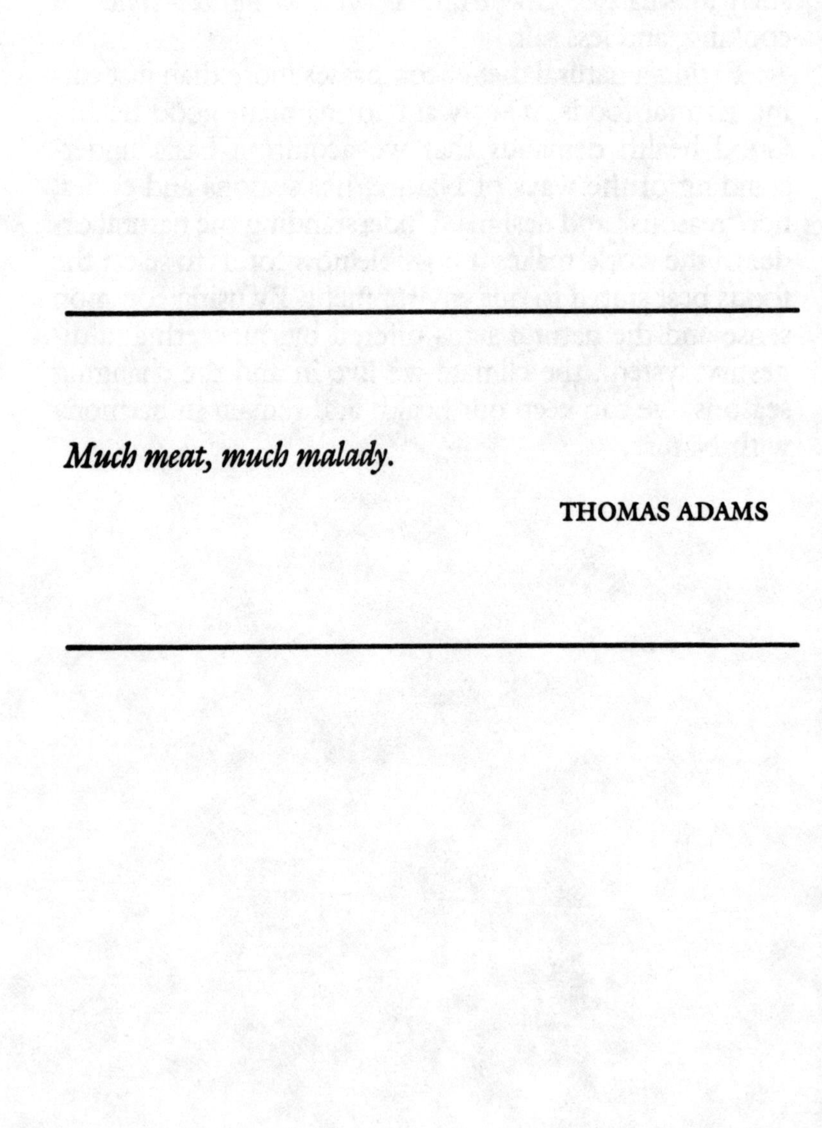

Much meat, much malady.

THOMAS ADAMS

Foods To Avoid

Meat

When looking at the practice of eating meat from a large (i.e., macro) perspective, we can see that it is the eating of a "related" species. In other words, it is the eating of *other mammals* like ourselves, which makes it a kind of 'cousin cannibalism'. Societies that nourish themselves in this way tend to develop, as a whole, a more aggressive, 'predatory' outlook, whereas cultures that abstain from meat tend to be more peaceful.[25] Since human beings are already basically quite yang (i.e. highly active and organized) it is wiser to balance this yang nature with more yin foods—foods which come primarily from the plant kingdom rather than from the animal kingdom. When we eat animals (which are very yang) we become, as a result, too yang ourselves. This can manifest *individually*—(meat eaters, as a whole, tend to be more quarrelsome or domineering than grain eaters) or *collectively*—(meat-eating countries tend to politically dominate, militarily conquer or economically exploit other countries). Excessive consumption of meat may well be the main reason for war and bloodshed throughout history.

The effects of eating violently killed creatures can be harmful in other ways as well. As Peter Forrest states in his article *Slaughterhouse*—"I have seen first hand what goes down when animals are butchered, strung up on hooks and torn apart by an incredibly inhumane process . . . simply because the blood and life is gone from a carcass does not mean the tension, the terror and the adrenalin are gone also . . . when you eat the flesh of any animal that has been butchered violently, you are eating fear, you are eating terror and all the hormones which accompany terror."

Throughout history many great men discovered the deleterious effects produced by meat-eating and chose to refrain from this practice. Plato, Plutarch, Ovid, Seneca, Diogenes, Milton, Pope, Shelley, Voltaire, Rousseau, Thoreau, Tolstoy, Newton, Gandhi and G. B. Shaw were some of the men who perceived the ill effects of meat and excluded it from their diet. As well, Trappist, Buddhist and Carthusian monks among other religious orders, also eat vegetarian diets which more easily support a spiritual outlook and aid in bringing peace and calm to the mind. Many of these vegetarians throughout history have been on the 'right track' so to speak, but they have lacked a deep, comprehensive understanding of the overall dietary principle involved and were thus unable to explain their instinctive preference to others in a complete and effective way.

Lastly, among people who consume considerable quantities of meat, there is often a physical resemblance imparted by these foods to those who ingest them, which can range anywhere from mild to severe. Due to the increased, and now excessive, consumption of meat in our culture, it is now a common sight to observe individuals with a 'beefy' look about them, or occasionally one with distinctly pork-like features, an indication that by eating meat we are regressing back towards lower forms of life instead of evolving towards a higher one.[26] Fortunately, these unpleasant attributes can fade in time by eliminating these unsuitable foods from our diet and by replacing them with healthful, natural wholefoods.

Fish are an acceptable food in the macrobiotic diet because fish live in a water environment, a factor which makes them much less yang than mammals or fowl. Water is a yang element, being heavier and more dense than air. To survive in such a specialized yang environment fish adapt by becoming more yin. However, due to their *active* nature they are still more yang than plants. But when animal protein is desired or where it is required due to heavy physical labor, fish is a less extreme choice than meat and a much better source of animal protein, in moderate quantities of course. However, there are variations among fish, some being relatively more yang and some being relatively less yang. Those which are slow-moving and which have white flesh are more moderate, while those which are very active or which have red flesh are very yang and are best avoided, as indicated on the food-classification chart.

Dairy Foods

To the people of many countries, our custom of drinking milk and eating cheese and butter is perceived as strange and eccentric behavior. Though a very familiar habit to us, if we look at this practice for a moment from another angle, we may be able to understand that it is entirely outside the realm of commonsense and natural order; for no other animal in the world gives the milk of another species to its young to drink, as do we. We reroute the milk of cows (a substance intended by Nature to create the body and brain of a cow) to our children. This may be why many American children have gradually assumed slightly bovine characteristics in recent decades during which time there has been a great increase in dairy food consumption. Many of them are beginning to develop the passive attitudes, sluggish movements and dull countenances so characteristic of cows. In this sense they are becoming the "foster children" of cows. But so ingrained is this practice in our culture, that we have become mesmerized and do not perceive it as at all abnormal.

In addition, all other mammals in nature *cease* nursing their young after the time of infancy. We, however, do not. We continue to 'nurse' even as adults, by drinking milk and indirectly by eating milk products, such as ice cream and cheese. And though we know that, as children grow, their lactase level naturally goes down (lactase being the intestinal enzyme used by the body to digest lactose, the main carbohydrate in milk) our present-day thinking is so upside down that some of our leading nutritionists do not look upon this change as part of a natural development *signalling that infancy has terminated,* but rather consider it, oddly, 'an inherited condition'.

The practice of eating dairy foods is very addictive, however, and most people find it easier to gradually replace dairy products with tasty substitutions similar in texture and type (such as tofu 'cheeses', nut-butter creams, almond milk, and soy milk, etc.) In time, the body begins to draw on other, more beneficial sources of nutrients, as we 'evolve' from a dairy food diet—to temporary substitutions—to a normal dairy-free macrobiotic diet.

Sugar

There is little good to say about sugar, whether the subject is white sugar, brown sugar, raw sugar, turbinado sugar, or any other variety. Much literature abounds, however, on the *ill* effects of this foodless food[27]—on the multitude of ways that it rots the teeth, dims the eyesight, causes acne, thins the blood, dulls the hair and weakens the bones. It is also becoming known as the culprit that causes depression, confusion, despondency and even senility—robbing us, year by year, of our natural birthright of robust health and high spirits.

As addictive as some drugs, sugar has crept into almost every kind of packaged and processed food on the market under various names and disguises. It is now included not only in foods such as cookies and cakes, but also in our bread, soups, vegetables, sauces and even in our salt. In fact, few foods can be found that are free of this harmful substance that so thoroughly saturates our modern diet.

What happens to healthy societies when sugar is introduced clearly shows its pathological effects. But force of habit, addiction, and 'sugar-coated' advertising have kept us consuming our daily doses of this slow-working poison. Sugar is an extremely yin food (tropical in origin, extremely sweet in taste and highly refined and processed) consisting of concentrated and potent crystals whose 'pure' appearance belies their destructive force.

When a society such as ours experiences decay from within (evident in America's alarming increase in cancer and heart disease rates and other degenerative ailments) the first step it must take towards rejuvenating the health of its citizens is to eliminate sugar from its diet. For, aside from drugs and alcohol, no other habitually consumed substance is as powerful as sugar in its ability to erode the health of a nation. More wholesome sweeteners can be used to provide a sweet taste, such as barley malt, maple syrup, rice syrup, fruit juices and fruit concentrates, most of which are available at any good natural food store.

Tropical Fruits

With their soft or watery pulp, which bruises and decomposes easily, these extremely yin fruits impart their own characteristics to those who eat them, i.e. their swollen, puffy flesh and weak natures. Mangoes, papayas, bananas and certain melons (as well as other tropical fruits) can eventually weaken our health if we take them frequently.

In addition, many of these fruits have been so overcultivated and hybridized that they are much different than those which are left to grow naturally—another factor which further weakens and distorts their qualities. Fruit trees, for instance, which have not been tampered with, tend to produce smaller (less yin) fruits, rather than the overblown, expanded (very yin) fruits now being artificially grown.

Even subtropical fruits such as oranges and grapefruits are not appropriate to eat more than very occasionally. Their many yin characteristics indicate that they are an extreme food, and that they will therefore eventually create an extremely yin condition in our bodies.

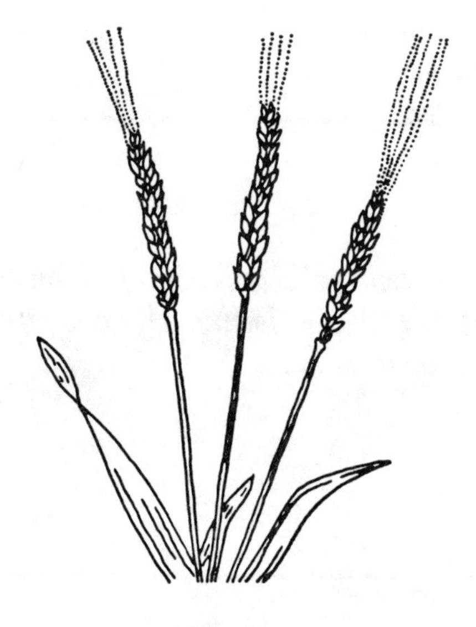

Wheat

............true balance is not a position of rigidity, but one of great ease.....a flowing with every moment, giving, taking, adjusting.......

THE DEVAS

More About Yin and Yang

As stated, it was traditionally understood in the Orient that everything in Nature, not only food, is influenced by yin and yang. Since all phenomena are affected by these two kinds of energy, we can evaluate anything in Nature to determine which influence predominates.

Observing the seasons of the year, summer is yang, for it is very hot, sunny and bright with foliage in full bloom. Winter is the opposite, yin, characterized by colder, darker days (or less sunshine)—an inward, hibernating time of year. Spring and fall are transitional periods between these two opposite poles which rotate back and forth in a continual cycle. Night and day present another example. During the day it is bright and much warmer than nightime, that is to say, it is yang. Night transforms into the opposite—a time of dark and cold, i.e. yin. Dawn and twilight are periods of transition between the two, again rotating in a continual cycle of change.

The plant and animal kingdoms provide still another example of yin and yang. Animals, as a whole, are active and warm-blooded—chasing, flying, jumping, barking and buzzing—all yang activities. Plants, on the other hand, are cool, silent and stationary; in other words they are more yin. In observing the human race we see, again, yin and yang. Men are generally more yang, meaning that they are more assertive, more active and outgoing in personality and that they possess harder, stronger bodies. Women on the whole are more yin, meaning that they are generally more gentle and sympathetic in attitude and that they possess softer, more sensitive bodies.

These are only a few simple examples of how Nature consists of two contrasting opposites, whatever aspect of the world we choose to look at. Chemistry, physics, biology and even art, music and history all offer examples of yin and yang as does every other manifestation of Nature or expression of humanity. Perceiving these two opposites in life or Nature provides endless interest as well as a game which even children can enjoy. But at the same time, the mechanism of how these two opposites act and interact can be a delicate and subtle riddle occupying the efforts of the most astute thinkers. Since yin and yang are not fixed states, but constantly change from one into the other (sometimes at a very slow rate, sometimes more rapidly) the study of this flux or cycle traditionally absorbed the attentions of Oriental scholars.

This understanding of yin and yang can now be applied in our modern world to solve problems in fields ranging from agriculture to technology, and to better understand in general the world we live in. A basic comprehension of yin and yang—and the principles of their interaction—is like a prism that differentiates into different purposes and significance according to the angle of our perceptions; once its value is fully grasped, humanity will diffuse this understanding into a hundred thousand uses and purposes.

Variations Within A Category

The more we know about yin and yang, the better we can understand how they work. One important point is that there are many shades or gradations of yin and yang, not just a few static categories. On the chart we see that sugar (and this means any food containing sugar as well) is extremely yin, for sugar is very sweet, grows very tall or large, and originates in a tropical climate—all very yin characteristics. In addition, it is highly refined, which adds still another yin influence. Therefore, foods which contain sugar have very yin expansive effects; they tend to produce a swollen or weak condition in the body's tissues and organs and, as previously mentioned, they can make us mentally confused or depressed. Also on the chart we can see that another unbalanced food is meat—positioned at the other end of the spectrum. Meat is very yang as we have seen, , for animals are very active and warm-blooded. Their flesh, when eaten, tends to produce a contracted or overly tight condition in the body's tissues and organs. Mentally, meat can also produce an oppressive 'heavy' feeling, or even an aggressive, restless or irritable attitude.

However, this food-classification chart shows only the relative yin-to-yang classification of different kinds of foods. In addition to this general classification there is also a more subtle range of yin and yang *within each category* of foods. For instance, taking the category of fruits, which as a whole are yin, because they are sweet, juicy, rich in potassium, etc.—there are some fruits which are more yin and some which are less yin. This is because not all fruits have exactly the same qualities. Some are larger like grapefruit (more yin) while others are smaller like cherries (less yin). Some grow in tropical or sub-tropical climates like pineapples (more yin) while others can grow in temperate climates like strawberries (less yin). These and many other factors help us to compare the various qualities of fruits or other foods to determine whether they are more extreme types or more moderate types. As a result, we can understand why certain foods are safe to consume, while others are less so . . . why one fruit is acceptable, while another is not . . . why one kind of fish is recommended while another is best avoided. We can best understand this reasoning when we observe as many qualities of a food as possible.

In the following comparison of two fruits, we can see that one possesses more moderate qualities, while the other possesses qualities that indicate it is too extreme to consume on a regular basis. This can be seen only by looking carefully at each fruit's individual characteristics. (See chart at right).

By more closely observing the various qualities of these two fruits it becomes clear that though apples are yin (sweet, juicy, containing potassium, etc.) they are less yin than bananas. Thus apples may be more safely consumed on a regular basis, while bananas would tend to produce very yin effects in our bodies if eaten regularly. This range of yin and yang—*this variation within a category*—appears in *all* food groups. Another example may be seen in the vegetable category. While most vegetables are classified in the more balanced or more moderate range, there are several vegetables which possess extreme qualities and which are, therefore, not recommended. These include those belonging to the night-shade family—such as potatoes, eggplant and tomatoes—which are extremely rich in potassium and tropical in origin. However, as a general category, vegetables and all other *food*

	BANANAS	APPLES
SHAPE	Bananas have an *elongated,* linear shape (more yin).	Apples have a more *round* and compact shape (less yin).
SKIN	Bananas have skins which are *loose* and easily separated from the fruit (more yin).	Apples have skins which adhere *tightly* to the fruit (less yin).
DENSITY	The fruit of a banana is very *soft* and easily bruised (more yin).	The fruit of apples is more dense and *hard* (less yin).
CLIMATE	Bananas need a *warm,* comfortable *climate* to survive (more yin).	Apples are more hardy and can thrive in *colder climates* (less yin).
POTASSIUM CONTENT	Bananas are very *rich in potassium* (more yin).	Apples contain *less potassium* (less yin).
STORAGE	Bananas begin to *decompose* within a relatively short period of time (more yin).	Apples can *store* well for long periods of time, for weeks and even months (less yin).

groups are classified in their approximate range relative to each other and relative to their appropriateness for daily consumption. While it is not necessary to know the varying degrees of each and every food, it is important to know which foods of any food group are not beneficial for our health, such as tropical fruits or nuts and certain kinds of fish and vegetables as shown on the food-classification chart.

Not Fixed States

Though for general purposes it is unnecessary to analyze foods so minutely, it is also important to understand that yin and yang are not fixed states, but change according to circumstances. To understand this point we may take the comparison of yin and yang a step further by looking at two of the same kind of foods. For even two of the same foods will vary in their yin or yang qualities. Using the example of carrots, we can see that no two carrots are exactly alike and that yin and yang are changing states reflecting many varying factors. Carrots grown by one farmer, for instance, may have been sprayed with pesticides and fumigants, which are yin, while carrots grown by another farmer may have been grown organically without the use of these yin substances, making them relatively more yang. The first carrots may have been over-watered (yin) causing them to swell and crack or rot more quickly, while the second carrots may have received only rainfall or minimal irrigation (more yang). Some vegetables are now grown hydroponically, that is, in water with nutritional supplements added (again yin), while others are allowed to grow naturally in the earth (more yang). These variations in the growing process influence the quality of foods accordingly, making them either more yin or more yang. While it is preferable to obtain good organic produce whenever possible[28], it is not necessary to become overly concerned about these points. However, it is important to understand, as just illustrated, that since many different influences go into creating any particular food, the variations in these influences such as climate, amount of irrigation, growing season, quality of the soil, etc. will produce changes either more yin or more yang. This demonstrates that yin and yang are not *static* conditions but that they can be altered in degree and quality by various factors.

Even if we know nothing about yin and yang these various influences are apparent. In some parts of the world where modern agri-business has not reached, the fruits sold in the markets are often less perfect to the eye than those sold in ultra-modern supermarkets. They are often smaller, they may have blemishes, and they are not waxed, fumigated or sprayed. But their flavor is incomparable, full and rich. The American apple or pear, on the other hand, may be bigger and it may be more beautiful with its waxy shine and individual bed of colored tissue, but it is often a disappointing, tasteless texture of overblown fiber, pumped up with chemicals and water. The same holds true for many vegetables such as cucumbers, sweet corn and squash which often possess only a faint flavor, reminiscent of what should be their actual taste. To deal with this problem, many cooks increasingly add sugar, spices and monosodium glutamate (MSG) to 'enhance' foods—which really means to make up for the natural flavors missing from so many of our foods.

In a sense the American farmer and the American consumer have become partners in a self-defeating alliance. The farmer pumps up his produce with chemical stimulants, motivated more by profit than quality, while the consumer insists on picture-perfect produce, offended in his artificial environment by any taint of earth or insect on his fruits and vegetables. Unfortunately this unspoken pact has sacrificed the quality of our fruits, grains, and vegetables (and thus our health) for the sake of appearance and profit.

Altering Foods Through Cooking

Another consideration is that the yin or yang quality of a food can be modified to some degree depending on how it is prepared in the kitchen. Salt has traditionally been used by many cultures to offset the somewhat yin 'rawness' of uncooked vegetables, thus transforming them into pickles, a process which attempts to balance (or lightly yangize) the raw (yin) state, while still retaining the freshness of an uncooked vegetable. Fire, also yang, is another factor which is used to alter the original properties of foods.

Certain yang foods are occasionally eaten in their raw or yin state. Cooking would render their already yang nature more yang. Thus the Japanese and Eskimoes often eat fish, particularly the more yang varieties, in a more yin (raw) form. This is only one example of the instinct for balance to be found in traditional cultures.

So, by roasting, drying, steaming, baking, pickling, etc. the original properties of a food can be modified to some degree. Therefore, raw foods and cooked foods have very different effects on us due to the change in quality that arises through the process of cooking and through the addition of such factors as salt, oil, water and so forth. Both raw and cooked foods are beneficial when included in a varied diet, but neither should be eaten exclusively. This would result in a diet either too yin (all raw) or too yang (all cooked).

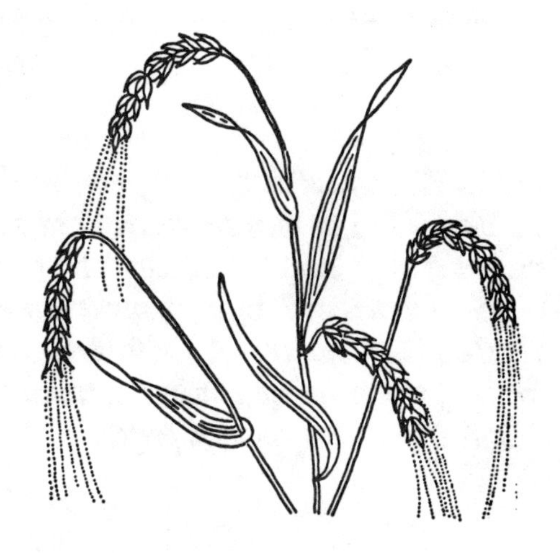

Barley

The word "macrobiotics" is derived from Greek and comes from a phrase in Hippocrates where he says that life is short but the art is long, ho bios brachys, hē techrē makre. Macro *combines with* bios, *to make macrobiotics, which means the art of long life. A Latin derived word could be "prolongevity", the meaning of which is much the same, but macrobiotics is the word that we prefer."*

JOSEPH NEEDHAM
Comparative Macrobiotics
Science in Traditional China

Defining Macrobiotics

Macrobiotics is many things to many people.

For most it is a natural lifestyle and healthy diet, and a way to make a living while contributing to the health and welfare of others; for those who seek self-development, it is a tool that promotes physical strength and mental clarity; for the curious and questioning, it opens up a world of fascinating possibilities—a new and unlimited science with ancient roots; for the fashion-conscious, it is a beauty aid and a way of staying slim; for the compassionate and the caring, it is a solution to the problem of world hunger; for the profit-minded, it is a budding industry with indications of a strong future; for the desperate and dying, it is precious lifeboat and a reprieve from the death sentence; for seekers of truth, it is a means to an end; for opportunists, it is a bandwagon and one more way to take advantage; for the selfless, it is a way to relieve the sick and the suffering of their misery; and for dreamers of things to be, it is the harbinger of a golden age.

Obviously a definition of macrobiotics is not easily arrived at, due to the many ways it can be perceived or utilized. Just as difficult is an attempt to cover, in a single definition, the many subjects included within its scope. For the study of macrobiotics is the study of the entire universe because it is the study of yin and yang—the basic principle or law of Nature. Macrobiotics is actually a branch (or, more accurately, a tree) of knowledge still under development and, considering its limitless aspect, it shall probably always remain so, as long as human beings want to know more about themselves and their world. But to gain some perspective on this unique way of thinking or unique principle as it is sometimes called, it is necessary to, at least, attempt a definition of this all-encompassing understanding of life and Nature.

A WAY OF LIFE

Macrobiotics is a natural way of living, a composite of healthful living practices based mainly on a diet of wholefoods. It also includes the wearing of natural-fiber clothing, regular exercise, and thorough chewing of one's foods. Additionally, it promotes an attitude of respect for Nature and careful use of the earth's resources.

A PRINCIPLE

Macrobiotics is the study and application of the principle of yin and yang, not only to the area of diet and health, but to all other aspects of Nature and life as well. This principle is known as the Unifying principle, since it unifies all opposites in the world by perceiving them as opposite sides of a single whole. East and West, analytical and wholistic, ancient and modern . . . these and all other contrasting phenomena are viewed as complementary opposites, none excluded or denied, all accepted and recognized.

A DREAM

The value of this unified perspective is its potential to foster a broader outlook on the world, an acceptance of other cultures, ways of thinking and kinds of people. This, in turn, can help bring about a better understanding between people from different countries. Within macrobiotic educational efforts a goal has been set. This goal (or dream, as it is sometimes called) is the realization of world peace, in its fullest sense; not only the cessation of needless human suffering and death through war, but also a true peace born of a common understanding among people who share life together on earth.

Defining a Macrobiotic Diet

A macrobiotic diet, in itself, is only one example of the way yin and yang can be applied for the benefit of mankind. There are also many ways, however, of defining the macrobiotic diet.

A NATURAL FOOD DIET

A macrobiotic diet is composed of foods which are naturally grown (without the use of chemicals, sprays, and fumigants, etc.) and which are used, as much as possible, in their natural state (unrefined and unprocessed).[29] The difference between a macrobiotic natural-food diet and other natural-food diets is that in a macrobiotic diet these natural foods are not selected at random, but according to a principle, the principle of yin and yang.

A WHOLEFOODS DIET

In a macrobiotic diet wholefoods are used rather than partial foods. Thus carrots are used in their entirety—the nutritious green tops as well as the orange roots; whole-wheat flour which retains the bran, rather than white flour, from which the bran has been removed; whole brown rice vs. polished white rice; the skin of an apple as well as its inner fruit, and so forth. In other words, in a macrobiotic diet foods are utilized the way Nature made them.

A REGIONAL DIET

A macrobiotic diet is also based as much as possible on regional foods, especially with regard to fruits and vegetables. This preserves the harmony between plants and environment that automatically develops in any particular region, a harmony that should be reflected in our diet. However, in the absence of regional foods, as is often the case today, foods brought in from a similar type of climate are recommended.

A TRADITIONAL DIET

A macrobiotic diet is also patterned on the time-honored custom, in many parts of the world, of consuming grain as the central or principal food. Supplemental foods have traditionally consisted, in varying combinations, of animal proteins, vegetable proteins, seeds, nuts, vegetables, fruits and dairy foods.

A WHOLISTIC DIET

A macrobiotic diet is a wholistic way of eating for it not only helps to maintain physical health, but it also promotes the development of a clear mentality and sound emotions. By taking into account the effects of foods on *all* aspects of our being, a macrobiotic diet helps us gain control of our lives and gives us the key to understanding our own nature.

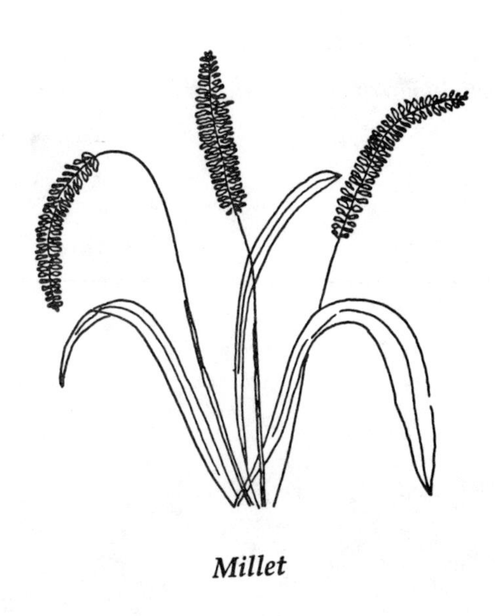

Millet

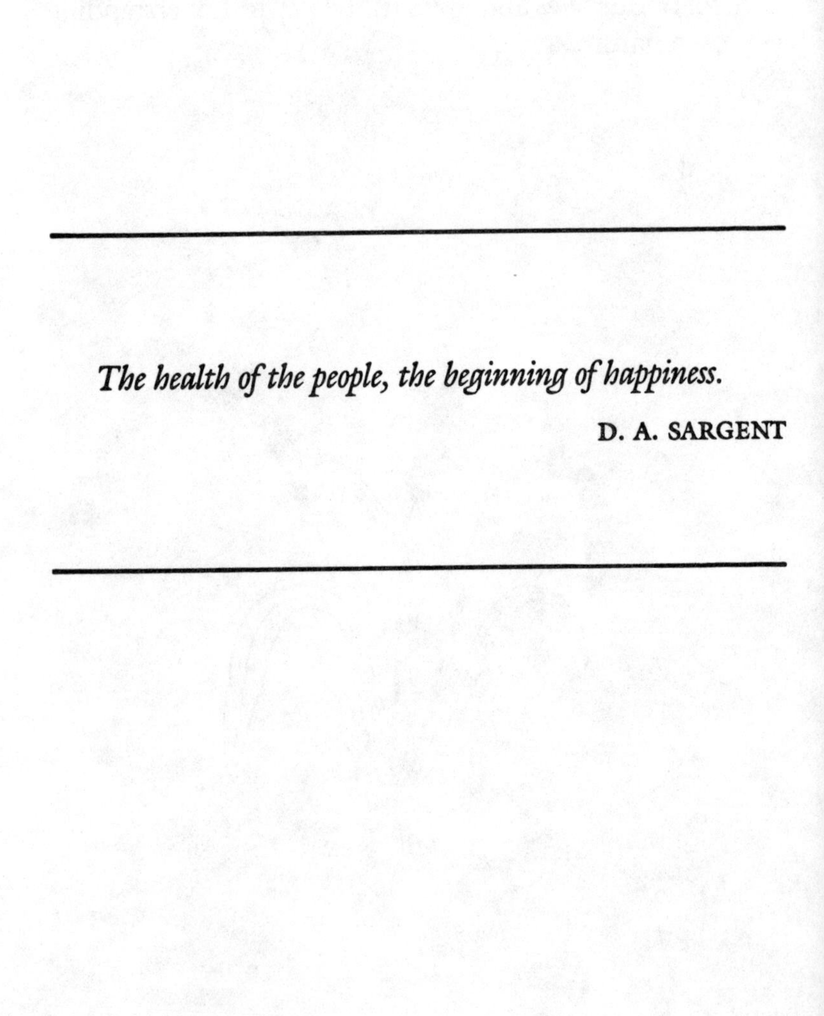

The health of the people, the beginning of happiness.

D. A. SARGENT

An Overview of Food

Foods affect much more than our health. So deeply do they influence us that they can even alter our attitudes and shape our ideas. Two striking examples of dietary influence may be seen in the lives of Adolf Hitler and Mahatma Gandhi. Hitler combined in his personality the aggression produced by excessive quantities of meat in his early life with the crazed mentality that results from excessive sugar consumption. He regularly consumed two pounds of chocolate per day and had only four of his own teeth left in his mouth. His life and attitudes were nothing more than a very extreme example of cause and effect, when viewed from the macrobiotic perspective. So deranged a mind as his was a predictable consequence of the disordered and extremely unbalanced diet that he consumed.[30]

A second example of dietary influence in the life of a historical figure may be seen in the life of Mahatma Gandhi.[31] Gandhi's parents were strict orthodox Hindus, to whom meat-eating (including eggs) was abhorrent. A life-long vegetarian, Gandhi developed the idea of *Satyagraha* or peaceful defiance of government. He led a strong, but non-violent, campaign to win independence for his country, and he was saddened when his followers sometimes turned to violence.

Another improper use of food, and its consequence, can be seen in the excessive use of spices in some parts of the world. Spices—strong stimulants—were traditionally known in Japan for their tendency to produce a discordant mental state. Buddhist monks, aware of this effect, avoided the use of spices in their cooking since the consumption of spiced food was disruptive to the attainment of a calm state of mind. In some areas of the world, food is often heavily spiced, a factor which may at least contribute to the unstable political and social climates in many of these regions. The examples utilized here are extreme ones, of course, which demonstrate the influence of food most clearly.

Nearly every nation affords a rich study in the relation between its diet and its physical and mental characteristics, and even its morals, attitudes and customs. The Japanese diet, a light one of rice, fish and vegetables, (though somewhat deteriorating in recent years due to the introduction of Western foods) still remains among the best in the world, permitting the Japanese to enjoy a society of high productivity, a very high rate of literacy, low crime and dignified aging, a correlation well worth America's attention and investigation.

When in some future age we have achieved a thorough understanding of food and its power, we will be far more capable of understanding the variations that arise in human nature. According to the macrobiotic view, food is the largest single factor controlling human destiny. Thus, by studying the food patterns of different societies, as well as those of various groups within a society, and by researching the food preferences of specific historical individuals, we may eventually come to understand the rhyme and reason of history.

Little can be accomplished in the struggle for racial harmony when minds are locked into rigid ideas and feelings of superiority by excessive quantities of meat, eggs or salt. Little ground can be gained in the fight against illiteracy when children's minds have been deactivated and dulled by non-nutritious donuts and empty, sugar-coated cereals. Eventually we will arrive at the realization that we, as individuals, *largely control our lives*—i.e. the quality of our physical health and mental outlook—*by what we choose to eat.*

Gradually we must understand that food has other effects on us besides that of fueling our bodies. We know that eating is the most basic concern of any form of life, the one which precedes all others. But it is also the oldest of rituals. When a family eats the same foods together year after year, and in some places generation after generation, there develops the binding force of similar body chemistry and similar outlook on life which develops and preserves a bond of understanding and agreement. Eating together, especially when the meals are of a wholesome quality, can maintain family unity and help create a common understanding among family members, and often a common work in life as well.

On a larger scale, this same principle applies. By eating similar foods, different countries, cultures and races can more readily understand one another. They can more easily sense a kinship instead of the separateness with which many individuals now perceive 'foreigners'. The latter attitude leads to fear and distrust and is fostered by vastly different eating patterns, which produce conflicting values and points of view. Whatever cultural variations arise from differences in climate, tradition, environment, religion, government, education and so forth, if people consume grain in any one of its many forms as their principal food *this factor alone,* in the macrobiotic view, is capable of creating a shared understanding and an ability to see our basic oneness rather than our minor differences. From this large or 'macro' view the common food of grain is the key to a common understanding. Therefore, restoring dietary order to the world can be the bridge that closes the gap, and in some cases, the chasm between nations.

From this perspective we can also see that by decreasing our dependence on meat and other animal proteins we can also reduce the urge of various nations to conquer and dominate each other (politically, religiously, or economically) and thus give ourselves a better chance for a peaceful co-existence. But this freedom can only come if we interrupt the existing cycle of cause and effect (meat and aggression, meat and racial discord, etc.) and learn how to control *that which controls us*—our food.

Macrobiotics holds aloft the hope that as the nations of the world learn how food sways and influences their behavior and attitudes, and as they develop more healthful and peaceful attitudes that arise from a wholesome diet—that from this simple but solid foundation of health, world peace will slowly, but surely, grow.

It would be foolish, of course, to think a day might ever come when peaceful coexistence will be a simple matter. In any era, no doubt, it will remain a complex quest, requiring serious exertion, patience and compromise on the part of all nations. But dietary change *can* pave the way for these other efforts, which may otherwise be futile endeavors. So though a healthful diet may not be the only answer to the goal of world peace, it can be the fundamental base on which to build. Clearly, a rush to embrace dietary change as a panacea for any and all problems would be simple-minded and naive. But conversely, to underestimate food and the tremendous power it has to shape our collective future is to be far worse than naive, it is to obstruct the future happiness of all mankind.

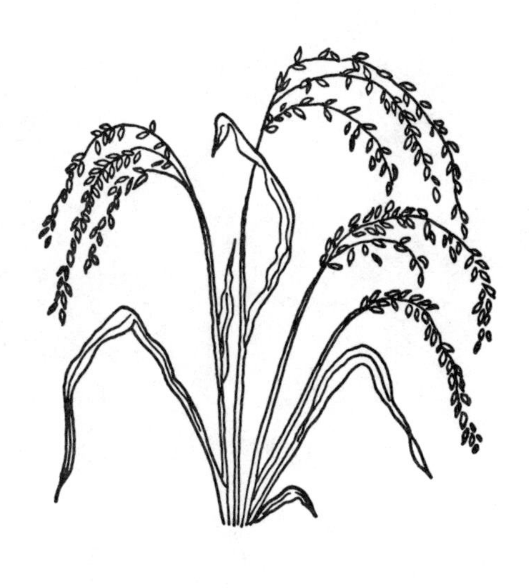

Rice

APPENDIX

When history is in the making, it is often difficult for those who witness it to assess events clearly. So close is their seat to the drama that often they lack an objective perspective—for objectivity is generally granted only by distance and time. Though not much more than a decade has passed since I first learned about the macrobiotic way of health, there has been time enough to acquire more than just a passing acquaintance with its principles and practice. This may be an insignificant period when measured on a grander scale of time; but it affords a better view than that seen by those who, freshly encountering so large a subject, struggle to find its boundaries and establish its limitations. But these boundaries do not exist, for macrobiotics is not a finite study, but an endless reading of the riddle of the universe. What we know about its history, however, may at least be recorded. Therefore, the following is offered as a short review of macrobiotic development—a brief look at the roots of this deep and long overdue change underway in our society, a change which is only now just beginning.

Origins

The very earliest origins of macrobiotics, or rather, the very earliest origins of the study of yin and yang, are obscured in the distant past. We know that prior to the time of Confucious and Lao Tzu (approx. 600 to 500 B.C.) there was a period in Chinese history known as the CHO dynasty. This was preceded by the YIN dynasty, which was further preceded by the archeologically remote KA dynasty. Prior to the KA dynasty, in a relatively unknown epoch, there was what is known as the Age of the Three Emperors—Fu-Hi, Shin-Noh and the "Yellow Emperor". Legend has it that these are the three who taught and developed the basic principles of yin and yang.

It is thought that Fu-Hi was the originator of the cosmological concept of yin and yang; that he was the first to perceive and understand it sufficiently to develop the eight trigrams of the *I Ching,* from which the total sixty-four hexagrams were later derived. Shin-Noh is considered to be the first to have applied yin and yang to the study of diet, herbs and agriculture, while the "Yellow Emperor" was thought to have developed yin and yang in the area of medicine, acupuncture and social order. The writings that exist today are not, of course, directly from these three emperors, for there are no written texts from this distant age. It may be that these traditions were handed down in various ways and formulated into the existing texts, such as the *Yellow Emperor's Classic of Internal Medicine,* by later generations. Whether these three emperors really existed is not known; but, myth or not, the understanding of yin and yang still remains, whether originated by them or by others unknown.[32]

From these ancient beginnings, the study and use of yin and yang spread throughout the Far East, and underwent various developments. As is the case with any major body of knowledge, many streams and tributaries developed, until the use of yin and yang permeated Far Eastern cultures from the sciences to the arts. For centuries, countless teachers and interpreters applied these principles to fields as different as alchemy and physiognomy. But with the adoption of Western culture, much of what was known about these important principles was forgotten and lost. In Japan, for instance, their traditional medicine, which had been based on yin and yang, was scorned and officially replaced with Western medicine in their avid worship of all things scientific.

But though Japan abandoned its valuable heritage more than any other Asian country, when we consider the direct lineage of what is presently known as macrobiotics, it is the Japanese whom we must thank for having acted as the primary contributors to its development and preservation. Shyoeki Ando, Sontoku Ninomiya, Kenzo Futaki and especially Ekiken Kaibara are named in the *Book of Macrobiotics* as the "outstanding thinkers who advocated the spirit and practice of the macrobiotic way of life" from the 17th through the 20th century.[33] To these names we may also add Mizuno Nanboku and Manabu Nishibata. Without wishing to underestimate the very great contributions of those named above (which are beyond the scope of this brief book to properly acknowledge) it may be said that Sagen Ishizuka, George Ohsawa and Michio Kushi have constituted the three major links in the chain that was to eventually become the study of macrobiotics as we know it today.

In the latter part of the 19th century, Sagen Ishizuka (1850–1910), a member of the medical staff of the Japanese army, re-discovered the traditional yin-yang approach to health in an effort to cure a disease from which he suffered (that had not responded to modern Western medical treatment). From his discoveries, which he gleaned from ancient and classic texts, he created a diet that he called SHOKUYODO—or "The Way of Nourishment", concerning which he wrote several books. In his attempt to revive the use of this traditional way of healing, he applied modern terminology (alkaline and acid, sodium and potassium) rather than the traditional words of yin and yang. In this way he hoped to gain the interest of his countrymen who were at that time attuned only to that which was modern.

Ishizuka not only successfully treated himself with his diet but hundreds of other people as well, and he eventually gained recognition as one who could cure disease with food alone. He foresaw the immense potential an understanding of yin and yang could have for the world, particularly in the area of health. However, as neither his books nor any biography of him has yet been translated into English, very little detail about his life and work is directly available to the English speaking world.

In Ishizuka's footsteps followed Yukikazu Sakurazawa (1893–1966) who later took the name by which he is more commonly known—George Ohsawa. By some accounts[34] he had a tragic youth, but by others, a rather comfortable one. Until thoroughly researched, many points about Ohsawa's life also remain nebulous. But it seems to be certain, however, that he developed tuberculosis at a rather young age, and that after reading Ishizuka's book, he began practising the "Way of Nourishment" and did actually free himself of this disease.

Just as many of Ishizuka's theories were rooted in the findings of the generations that had preceded him, much of what Ohsawa eventually contributed to the development of macrobiotics was based on Ishizuka's work, as well as that of others. A diligent and industrious student, Ohsawa further systemitized Ishizuka's theories, and developed his own, slightly different, version of the ideal diet. The seven basic principles and twelve theorems that eventually composed the core of his teachings were gathered from traditional Oriental literature and then assembled by him in a cohesive and concentrated format.

In his attempts to introduce his teachings to the West (primarily in France and Belgium) he named his collective theories "Le Principe Unique"—(meaning the Prime or Superior Principle). He also selected the words "Order of the Universe" from classical writings to designate the laws of change at work in the universe, for he had by this time expanded his viewpoint beyond a medical or dietary application of yin and yang to the entire field of life itself. Adding still further to these (and many other) appellations, Ohsawa eventually chose the word macrobiotics to denote the study of yin and yang and the natural way of health. In the 1960's, towards the end of his life, he added the word "zen" to form Zen Macrobiotics, hoping with this appendage to generate more interest in his theories for the zen 'movement' was popular at that time.[35]

George Ohsawa's life and work were an invaluable, perhaps indispensable, bridge between Sagen Ishizuka and Michio Kushi, who was to become the next major teacher of the macrobiotic diet and principles. Ohsawa's eclectic mind, penetrating insight and pioneer spirit helped create what is becoming a major healthcare movement in the West. In addition, his remarkable ability to extract from traditional Oriental writings its most precious elements (i.e. the essence of universal order) mark him as an outstanding philosopher.

If Ohsawa did not directly succeed in awakening the world to his discoveries, he did succeed, at least, in awakening one who possibly could accomplish this feat—a young man by the name of Michio Kushi, in whom he immediately recognized a rare potential. Kushi's interest was world peace—the result, in part, of the horror he witnessed in World War II as a youth. Ohsawa urged him, quite determinedly, to undertake the study of yin and yang and diet as a means of establishing peace, for he understood that in a world where sickness prevails, there can be little hope of peace. His influence on Kushi may have been one of his greatest accomplishments, equal (in practical results) to his efforts in clearly focusing on the principles of natural law. For without Kushi, this knowledge might again have been lost with Ohsawa's death, except in a few unnoticed pockets of the world.

Though Ohsawa possessed an eccentric character, his very unique life and adventures, experiments and philosophy are a legacy which will someday earn him a place of distinction and honor in history. What may also be remembered about him is the great courage he showed in testing his discoveries and theories on himself.

On the deficit side, it may be seen that his interpretation of what are basically sound dietary principles was unfortunately highly stringent and rigid, far off-balance and incorrect for the vast majority of individuals.

Though some thousands of people benefited from his teachings (according to Kushi) most of his recommendations produce an overly yang or contracted state of mind and body, rather than a state of balanced health. This has caused many people to wisely abandon this version of a macrobiotic diet within a relatively short period of time. His interpretation was apparently also too extreme for himself as well; because though he cured his tuberculosis by altering his diet and lived decades beyond what was allotted him by modern doctors, he struggled ever afterwards with dietary extremes, particularly excessive salt. (His wife, Lima Ohsawa, who also cured her chronic ill-health[36] through macrobiotic dietary principles, was more moderate in her approach and continues to live a healthy active life in Japan, still teaching macrobiotic cooking, though she is well past the age of eighty. Her underestimated contribution as George Ohsawa's partner in his adventurous life has not yet been fully recorded.)

Ohsawa's writings, at least those which have been translated into English, are a strange amalgam of profound truths and preposterous boasts, wise advice and erroneous counsel. It takes a patient and discerning eye to distill the truth and beauty from these singular works. A man as unique as his principle, George Ohsawa is difficult to summarize. Tyrannical at times, he was also very humble; a fearless speaker of the truth, he also possessed an inclination towards fiction; he was belligerent yet introspective; a seeming fool to his contemporaries, but also something of a sage.

In recent years, however, it was Michio Kushi who vastly enlarged and developed the principles of yin and yang especially as they pertain to the study of humanity and its destiny. It is he, too, who is presently succeeding in introducing these valuable principles to Western nations, including their application to the areas of food, health and diagnosis.

Kushi, born in 1926, had initially displayed a lack of interest in Ohsawa's discoveries. Only after being prodded by Ohsawa's keen mind and piercing remarks did he undertake the study of yin and yang. After studying Ohsawa's and Ishizuka's works, and sifting through ancient texts, he began to further develop and apply yin and yang. His conclusion was that these were universal principles found East and West, North and South, throughout mankind's entire reach and history, not only within Oriental traditions. He, therefore, renamed the "Unique Principle" the "Unifying Principle" and later the "Universal Principle". He also simplified the seven principles of Ohsawa, and eventually discontinued the use of the word "Zen" which he considered a "limiting" term. Though not satisfied with the name "macrobiotics" he decided to continue its use until a better one could be found.

As Kushi modified and refined Ohsawa's work he also developed an enormous amount of original material independently, which will undoubtedly serve as an invaluable resource for generations to come. Though it is premature to assess his works, in view of the fact that they are still being produced, it is not premature to acknowledge that he had the stamina and fortitude to carry on through many stagnant and very difficult years in America before seeing any recognition of his work or fruits of his labor. A broad-minded man, of patient and gentle demeanor, his work is extraordinarily refined and of seemingly unlimited dimensions, unmatched for diversity and depth.

Though Ishizuka, Ohsawa and Kushi all contributed to the development of macrobiotics, each developed an outlook on society that influenced the scope of their teachings.[37] This may be due to the fact that each was influenced by different social conditions including the expanding development of transportation and communication systems, which may have successively broadened their views.

Ishizuka, in whose consciousness the spark linking ancient theories to modern uses first ignited, was primarily interested in medicine and health, and in enlightening his own countrymen with regard to his findings. He wanted to rekindle Japan's interest in its traditional medicine and dietary practices, for, as noted, Japan at that time had turned away from its native traditions in favor of things Western. A tireless, dedicated worker, Ishizuka lived and taught solely in Japan.

Ohsawa also defended this position, trying to interest his contemporaries in Japan's native traditions. But he also travelled to Europe, America and Africa (as a kind of self-appointed representative of Eastern philosophy) and even lived for many years in the West, though he continually returned to Japan to live and teach. In other countries Ohsawa always promoted the view that the East has merit as well as the West, and he carried the hope that the West would eventually come to recognize this fact. Though Japan-centered for much of his life he did widen his view to include a more universal application of his theories.

Kushi, however, detached himself from allegiance to any particular country, considering Japan to be "just one of many countries, no different from the rest". In the last thirty years, he has travelled extensively to many parts of the world, teaching the understanding of yin and yang, and seeking to raise the awareness of people from a national to a planetary level.

During Ohsawa's time, macrobiotics was not widely accepted, the result, perhaps, of two factors. First was

Ohsawa's considerably strict and inflexible dietary recommendations (which have been greatly modified by Kushi). It is not surprising that his highly rigid version of a basically sound diet was cause for alarm amongst the few doctors and nutritionists who encountered it.

Secondly, there was the further misuse of Ohsawa's already overly severe regimen by a few individuals, at least some of whom were involved with hallucinagenic drugs, substances which, from the macrobiotic view, suppress or inactivate one's instinctive common sense. As a result, macrobiotics gained a kind of vague reputation as an unsound diet, which indeed it was when so incorrectly taught or used. But this reputation is one that it is recently shedding, as people become educated to its more sensible and sound practice. This is why Kushi and other teachers have broadened and refined Ohsawa's original guidelines and increased the element of flexibility without which the macrobiotic diet cannot succeed.

With any new discovery or invention, the early years surrounding its 'birth' are usually fraught with problems, difficulties, imperfections and trial and error. This period usually redefines and reshapes the original knowledge more perfectly, and this has been the case with macrobiotics. And though Ohsawa may have given too severe and potentially dangerous recommendations due to the lack of time and further development of his teachings, still he and Ishizuka, and all those who preceded them, helped to carve a path through a very dense jungle of ignorance about diet, which permitted Kushi and others to enter and begin paving the way. Therefore, in spite of this deep defect—and perhaps it was not so much a defect as it was the lack of time and experience—it is not only to Kushi but also to Ohsawa, as well as to Ishizuka, that a great debt of gratitude is due.

So, the story of macrobiotics is essentially the story of

these three extraordinary men, and the host of others preceding them who served as their teachers. Each one carried the wisdom of these traditions foreward and outward, taking something from those who had gone before and giving back something of his own to those who came after.

Since each nourished the other, there is much duplication in their conclusions, and it would be difficult to draw the line as to where one's thinking stopped and the other's began. But such a line may not be necessary, for Orientals do not so much hold to the idea of an original creator or founder of a teaching. Rather they consider that some concepts or traditions were always existing throughout their race and that there are only various teachers, interpreters and practitioners who preserve and convey the wisdom from generation to generation.

The most recent major development to take place in the growth of macrobiotics has taken place through the efforts of Michio Kushi and his wife Aveline, (who has probably made the greatest contribution to educating Westerners in the art of macrobiotic cooking through the establishment of a macrobiotic cooking school). The Kushis have worked unceasingly to introduce the macrobiotic diet to people around the world. The difficulties they have jointly encountered in introducing the Eastern perspective[38] to the West have been immense. Yet it is mainly through their efforts that an understanding of food and its influence is at last being brought to America's attention.

Many of their students are continuing these efforts,[39] by establishing small educational centers where others in their community may go to learn more about macrobiotic nutrition. At this writing, many of these centers are in varying stages of development. Depending on the staff, the instruction available can range from excellent to inadequate. In an attempt to establish and maintain standards of excellence in macrobiotic education a certification program has been established by the Kushi Institute of Boston, Massachusetts, which serves as the main center for macrobiotic education in the United States.

But because the systemitized study of macrobiotics is still a very young one, only several years old, the number of qualified teachers in this field are still few. This is also due to the fact that macrobiotic nutritional counseling is an art which requires serious study of the different properties of a wide range of foods. The ability of counsellors depends on the depth and refinement of their understanding, a skill which takes much time and experience to acquire. So even those who have studied macrobiotics for years remain, in many ways, only novices. However, there are a number of very good macrobiotic centers throughout the United States, and Europe as well, which offer excellent instruction in macrobiotic cooking and dietary counseling. A current list of certified teachers and educational centers may be obtained from the Kushi Institute of Boston, Box 1100, Brookline, MA 02147.[40]

NOTES

1. Except with regard to deficiency conditions, and only in recent years with regard to cancer and heart disease. See, for example, *Diet, Nutrition and Cancer,* National Research Council, Washington, D.C., 1982 and *Dietary Goals for the United States,* Select Committee on Nutrition and Human Needs, United States Senate, 1977.
2. "In modern, conventional medicine the word 'cure' denotes the elimination of symptoms that do not reappear for a period of five years. However, in macrobiotics, there are two meanings to the word 'cure'. In a more limited sense it denotes a change in one's diet and lifestyle, from the course of degeneration and decline towards a healthy and sound dietary direction. In this sense the word 'cure' is used, though symptoms may still remain. They eventually disappear, however, through the continuation of a healthy diet and direction. But the real meaning of the word 'cure' in the macrobiotic sense is the achievement of total health. Total health includes both physical and psychological soundness, as well as freedom from all disorders, and further, an attitude of respect and love for Nature and all people. Ultimately, it includes the experience of a natural death (vs. death by disease or accident) and the unlimited development of consciousness".

   Michio Kushi
3. There are some conflicting viewpoints amongst various macrobiotic teachers on both major and minor points concerning macrobiotic thought. But the viewpoint referred to in this book is specifically that put forth by Michio Kushi, considered by this author to be the teacher with the clearest understanding and deepest comprehension of the subject. Unfortunately, only a

limited selection of his works have been published as of this writing.

4. Sagen Ishizuka, George Ohsawa, and Michio Kushi.
5. See *The Book of Macrobiotics,* M. Kushi, Japan Publications, 1977.
6. Such as atmospheric conditions, correct posture, the way we breathe, etc.
7. In Japan the traditional medicine which had been based on yin and yang was officially replaced with modern Western medicine.
8. As explained in *The Book of Macrobiotics,* M. Kushi, Chapter 1.
9. Except in the case of serious illness where even relatively minor dietary changes can produce a severe reaction.
10. There are cases where a person may temporarily subsist on a specialized diet (such as an exclusively fruitarian one) for a period of time, but in most cases, those who are attracted to eating this very yin type of diet are people who have previously eaten a very yang diet, heavy in meat, cheese or eggs. Thus, they are often trying to balance their former excessively yang diet by temporarily adopting an excessively yin one.
11. In this book the basic macrobiotic diet refers to the standard diet advised by Michio Kushi.
12. *Zen Macrobiotics,* George Ohsawa, Ohsawa Foundation, 1965—though this principle may have been adopted from Ishizuka's writings—or even earlier sources.
13. Obviously, education and family as well as other major influences play an important, crucial role in the mind's development. But according to macrobiotic principles, diet is, of all these, the most important influence.
14. *Why Your Child Is Hyperactive,* Ben E. Feingold, M.D., Random House, 1974.
15. *The Book of Macrobiotics,* M. Kushi, Japan Publications, *The Cancer Prevention Diet,* M. Kushi & Alex Jack, St. Martin's Press, *Natural Healing Through Macrobiotics,* M. Kushi, Japan Publications, *How To See Your Health,* M. Kushi, Japan Publication, etc.
16. The basic or original qualities of a food can be significantly altered during the cooking process, in such a way as to make them extreme.
17. *When eaten in sufficient variety, correctly cooked and not excessively seasoned.* See *Macrobiotic Dietary Recommendations,* The East-West Foundation, Boston, Massachusetts.

18. *The Book of Macrobiotics,* Composition of Foods Chart, M. Kushi, Japan Publications.
19. Except in very cold regions where grain does not grow, and where animal protein is required to balance the extreme climate.
20. Other foods containing salt (such as miso soypaste or tamari soy sauce) are also recommended as good quality seasonings; however, they should be used in moderation, never excessively, for excess salt can easily lead to an overly yang condition.
21. See *Macrobiotic Pregnancy and Care of the Newborn,* Michio and Aveline Kushi, Japan Publications, 1983.
22. The macrobiotic diet can include many other products, as well as foods used in other countries, with which we are only recently becoming acquainted, such as tofu, miso, tamari and tempeh. The *Natural Shopper's Guide* and *Macrobiotic Dietary Recommendations,* listed under "Recommended Reading" both offer more detailed information on macrobiotic natural foods of all kinds.
23. Michio Kushi, unpublished works.
24. Before the invention of modern food technology, people traditionally pickled vegetables or carefully stored the hardier varieties to eat over the winter months. Though these practices are excellent ones and highly recommended, they should not be relied upon solely as a source of vegetables during the winter season. This would constitute too abrupt and extreme a change, for we are unaccustomed to so limited and spartan a diet in winter. Therefore, in Northern temperate areas, it is recommended that during the colder months of the year, produce from temperate-range regions such as California or Florida be utilized, rather than produce from more distant tropical regions or the southern hemisphere.
25. However, excesses of other yang foods, not only meat, such as salt, eggs, or fish can also create an overly aggressive or cruel mentality.
26. We also see in recent years, more and more instances where women are developing physical characteristics similar to men due to the excessive consumption of meat, eggs and other very yang foods. As well, there are increasing instances where men are developing physical characteristics similar to women, due to excessive consumption of dairy foods, fruits, sugar products, and other very yin foods.

27. Such as *Sugar Blues,* William Dufty, Chilton Book Company, 1975; *Sweet and Dangerous—The new facts about the sugar you eat, as a cause of heart disease, diabetes and others killers,* I. Yudkin, P. H. Wyden, New York, 1972.

"That your health and your longevity are in a direct relationship to the *naturalness* of the foods you eat is a well-established scientific fact. Dr. Weston A Price, Vilhjalmur Steffansson, Dr. McCarrison, Arnold DeVries, and many others, who made extensive travels and studies of diet habits and their relation to health and longevity of practically every "primitive" people in the world, have found that when the diet was made of natural, fresh, unprocessed foods, grown in their own environment, the people had no disease or tooth decay. Conversely, where they discovered people subject to dental decay and various other degenerative diseases of civilized man, they invariably found that they ate denatured, cooked, processed foods, and that white flour, canned foods, and white sugar had made their way to them from more "civilized" countries. . . . .
"Arnold DeVries has studied the historical records of the North and South American Indians, Eskimos, Asians, Africans, Australian aborigines, New Zealand Maories, and people living on Pacific and Atlantic islands, and found that all of them enjoyed glowing health, great fertility and almost incredible endurance. Diseases were almost unknown. Women had fast and painless childbirths, and were usually back to their work in the fields an hour later. Men could run all day without fatigue. There was no tooth decay, or loss of sight or hearing, or gray hair. Although statistical life expectancy was low because of the poor sanitation, most of those who survived lived to be 100 years or over. DeVries also found that as soon as "civilized" foods were introduced to these people, their health began to decline. Childbirth became painful and prolonged; tooth decay made its impact; vitality and endurance abated; and they gradually became subject to all the diseases of "civilized" people."

by Paavo O. Airola, N.D. Ph.D.
Are You Confused
Health Plus, Publishers, 1981

28. There are not many foods on the market, at present, which are organically grown. Organic farming, however, is experiencing a

renaissance, and more organic produce is becoming available every year.

29. Except by traditional, non-chemicalized methods of processing, such as the transformation of soybeans into miso, tofu, tempeh, or tamari, etc.

30. Hitler considered himself a vegetarian later in life, but his diet included large quantities of eggs, which are more yang (or more unbalanced) than meat, since eggs are the most contracted, yang form of fowl. His cook apparently emphasized this element of his diet all the more because he was "vegetarian," and knew more than one hundred ways of preparing them. In addition, according to some biographies, Hitler often consumed pork in the form of pigs knuckles and sausage. Strangely, this did not alter his conviction that he was 'vegetarian'. The following excerpts offer some indication of his dietary extremes.

"He told one doctor that he had been a vegetarian since early youth, but to others he said that prior to 1931 he had eaten large quantities of meat, particularly fat'.

Adolf Hitler, The Psychopathic God
Robert G. I. Waite, Basic Books, Inc.

"The granddaughter of Richard Wagner remembered that, as a little girl, she and her sisters were fascinated by the amount of sugar and chocolates Hitler consumed while visiting their mother. He told them he ate two pounds of chocolates everyday. They waited expectantly for him to miscount the number of teaspoonfuls of sugar he invariably put in his tea, but he never miscalculated. Always there were seven. . . . . ."
(Hitler's) "ascetism was a fiction invented. . . . . to emphasize. . . . the distance that separated him from other men". ---- "in fact, he was remarkably self-indulgent and possessed none of the instincts of the ascetic." ----- "Although Hitler had no fondness for meat, except in the form of sausages, and never ate fish, he enjoyed caviar. He was a connoisseur of sweets. . . . . . which he consumed in astonishing quantities. He drank tea and coffee drowned in cream and sugar."

The Life and Death of Adolph Hitler
Robert Payne, Praeger Publishers, NY 1973

31. *The Life and Death is Mahatma Gandhi*, Robert Payne, Dutton, NY 1969.

32. Since any record of this development belongs to the realm of legend, many imaginary accounts have been created (in the same way that the story of Christ has been told in various fictionalized versions. Additionally, over the centuries many interpreters and commentators (often conflicting) have developed, including Confucious and King Wen. However, the modern macrobiotic interpretation of yin and yang by-passes these countless generations of interpreters and commentators and draws directly from Fu Hi's original concept of yin and yang.
33. These various teachers applied yin and yang to such different aspects of life and culture as Noh dance, tea ceremony, diet, physiognomy, martial arts and even flower arrangement.
34. Various accounts of Ishizuka and Ohsawa exist depending on which of his students relates their history. However, an investigation into the myths and facts is beyond the scope of this brief book.
35. As reflected in the writings of such authors as Suzuki and Alan Watts.
36. As related in the *Art of Just Cooking,* by Lima Ohsawa, published by Autumn Press.
37. In addition, Ohsawa and Kushi have both applied yin and yang to other areas besides diet, encompassing such subjects as history, chemistry, physics, agriculture, etc.
38. Eastern in the sense that the East is where this universal principle was most developed and applied.
39. Several 'schools' of macrobiotic thought have already developed, but some of these various tangents and outgrowths, while rooted in macrobiotic perspective, do not always necessarily express or reflect valid teachings, while others are making worthwhile contributions to our understanding of yin and yang.
40. This does not mean to imply that non-listed macrobiotic centers are unqualified to teach macrobiotics, nor even that all centers listed are unquestionably qualified. It is only to state that it is difficult to know which centers offer truly competent instruction from amongst the hundreds which exist, and that the certification program of the Kushi Institute is the best means presently available to locate a qualified counsellor in one's area.

Recommended Reading

GENERAL READING

Natural Healing Through Macrobiotics
by Michio Kushi, Japan Publications, 1978
How to See Your Health/Oriental Diagnosis
by Michio Kushi, Japan Publications, 1980
The Cancer Prevention Diet by Michio Kushi with Alex Jack, St. Martin's Press, 1983
The Natural Shopper's Guide by Dan Seamens and David Wollner, East West Journal, 1982
Macrobiotic Dietary Recommendations
by Michio Kushi, East-West Foundation, 1982
The East West Journal monthly magazine
Making the Transition to a Macrobiotic Diet by Carolyn Heidenry, Aladdin Press, 1984

COOKBOOKS

The Book of Wholemeals
by Annemarie Colbin, Ballantine Books, 1979
The Whole World Cookbook, International Macrobiotic Cuisine, Avery Publishing Group, 1984
National Foods Cookbook
by Mary Estella, Japan Publications, 1984
The Book of Tofu by William Shurtleff and Akiko Aoyagi, Ballantine Books, 1979
The Book of Tempeh by William Shurtleff and Akiko Aoyagi, Harper Colophon Books, 1979
The Sweet Life—Natural Macrobiotic Desserts
by Marcia Weber, Japan Publications, 1981